lorna sass' short-cut vegetarian

lorna sass'
short-cut
vegetarian

great taste in no time

QUILL

WILLIAM MORROW

new york

It is the policy of William Morrow and Company, Inc., and its imprints and affiliates, recognizing the importance of preserving what has been written, to print the books we publish on acid-free paper, and we exert our best efforts to that end.

Library of Congress Cataloging-in-Publication Data

Sass, Lorna J.
    Lorna Sass' short-cut vegetarian : great taste in no time / by
Lorna J. Sass.
        p.   cm.
    Includes index.
    ISBN 0-688-14599-X
    1. Vegetarian cookery. 2. Quick and easy cookery. I. Title.
TX837.S269   1997
641.5'636—dc21   96-48821
                                                          CIP

Printed in the United States of America

First Quill Edition

1 2 3 4 5 6 7 8 9 10

BOOK DESIGN AND ILLUSTRATION BY RICHARD ORIOLO

for richard

acknowledgments

Although writing and recipe development are primarily solitary pursuits, the efforts of many generous people are reflected in these pages. I extend heartfelt thanks to:

Rosemary Serviss, assistant extraordinaire, who offered delightful kitchen companionship throughout this project and contributed her considerable creative skill, especially to the breakfast and dessert chapters;

My many dear "elves" who cooked from the recipes, offered valuable suggestions for variations, and told me the real truth about prep times: Judy Bloom, Heather and Gerhard Boch, Munro Bonnell, Kay Bushnell, Evelyne Chemouny, Dena Cherenson, Arlene Ciroula, Joyce Curwin, Elizabeth Germain, Leigh Gibson, Erica Landis, Michelle Lunt, Maryann Mayo, Cathy Roberts, Tristan Roberts, Roberta Chopp Rothschild, Amy Schachter, Andrew Strauss, Sue Van Meter, Rachel Yurman, and Alisa Zlotnikoff. As with my previous books, Joan Carlton maintained her reputation of "super elf" by testing recipes just as fast as I could turn them out;

Those behind the scenes at William Morrow for making it all come together, including my editor Ann Bramson, senior editor Gail Kinn and assistant editor Jennifer Kaye, copyediting chief Deborah Weiss Geline and Judith Sutton for seeing to every last detail, and Richard Oriolo for the book's design;

Phyllis Wender, for agenting this book with such good cheer;

Susanne Speranza, for retyping the manuscript with such dispatch;

Eden Foods, Inc., for their generous contribution of superb organic ingredients for recipe testing;

Cliff Inkles and Ellen Oler for nourishing body and soul;

Elizabeth Schneider, for restorative walks, and Dorie Greenspan, for restorative talks; and

Richard Isaacson, to whom this book is dedicated, for scanning lost pages and making up for lost years.

contents

introduction

Once upon a time I believed in cooking everything from scratch. Then life got in the way.

Although I work at home—presumably the ideal circumstance for letting a pot simmer on the back of the stove—I began to find myself more and more frequently coming up against mealtime without a clue about what I'd be eating.

Pressure cooking—the subject of previous books—shortened cooking time dramatically, but still involved a fair amount of "schlepping and prepping" (aka "shopping and chopping"). Indeed, whenever I gave a lecture on vegetarian cooking or demonstrated one of my favorite lovingly prepared pressure cooker recipes, someone would invariably ask, "Is there any way to make really fast vegetarian food?"

As one who values eating fresh, wholesome vegetarian meals and considers chopping a form of meditation, I was reluctant to explore the question. But as the pace of life quickened, I found myself joining the growing number of cooks who search for ways to get dinner on the table more quickly.

I decided the first place to start was with a real staple of the vegetarian kitchen: dried beans. I love the taste of beans cooked from scratch, but they always take a bit of advanced planning because I prefer them presoaked. I was never happy with supermarket canned beans, since they are usually so salty and often contain preservatives. So I started, ever so cautiously, to experiment with organic canned beans from my local natural foods store.

I still remember the moment I opened that first can of organic red kidney beans. Sporting their gorgeous bold mahogany skins, these beans not only had great texture but also tasted good. Furthermore, the cooking liquid surrounding them was clear and low in sodium—no need to drain and rinse off any questionable substances.

The simple act of opening that can was a revelation—in fact, it awakened me to a whole new realm of quick-cooking culinary possibilities. If I, a hard-line "from scratch" cook felt good about keeping canned organic beans on hand, ready to prepare a last-minute chili or hummus, what other products and strategies might be available to harried cooks with high standards for quality, wholesomeness, and good taste?

Lorna Sass' Short-Cut Vegetarian offers you my hard-earned answers to that question. Writing this book has been an invigorating—often liberating—experience. Developing tasty, healthful vegan dishes (no dairy or eggs) that maximize flavor and good nutrition while minimizing preparation and cooking time has stretched my imagination and challenged me to enter realms previously unexplored.

I'm delighted to welcome you to *Lorna Sass' Short-Cut Vegetarian* kitchen, a place where very little effort produces substantial rewards. Happy cooking!

LORNA J. SASS
New York City

If you'd like to share your favorite short-cut recipes or strategies with me, or if you'd like advice on purchasing a pressure cooker, I'd be happy to hear from you. Please write to me c/o Cooking Under Pressure, Box 704, New York, NY 10024. Be sure to enclose a SASE if you want a response.

a few notes on using this book

necessity: the mother of great taste

I am a rebel in the kitchen and rarely cook a dish the same way twice. I may be running out of a particular spice or bean, or I may come upon a perfectly ripe vegetable screaming to be used. Any of these scenarios may end up transforming my original concept into something entirely new.

Since I am always thinking of different possibilities and new variations, I could not resist mentioning optional items in ingredient lists and recipe headnotes. These alternatives are intended to stimulate your imagination—but if you find them distracting or confusing, just ignore them and go straight to the basic recipe. I promise you that it will taste good as is.

Sometimes it's easier not to see all of the options. Believe me, I know. . . .

how many did you say it would serve?

To be honest, I'm not sure if my idea of a portion is the same as yours. Like most cookbook authors, I've struggled with the concept of serving size for years.

Just in case you find it helpful, I'd like to tell you that most people (not just my grandmother) think that I eat like a bird. If my serving estimates seem off to you, it's easy to make adjustments accordingly. Any of these recipes can be doubled or tripled for heartier appetites—or so you can freeze portions for meals down the road.

how I calculated prep time

My estimate of prep time is based on the number of minutes it takes to get the first group of ingredients into the pot. I have not included the time required for additional ingredients that can be prepared while the dish is cooking.

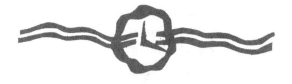

the short-cut

vegetarian kitchen

the short-cut vegetarian pantry

Stocking your kitchen with carefully selected high-quality canned, bottled, and dried ingredients is the first step to becoming a successful short-cut cook. Once you've assembled the basic items listed below, you'll be able to prepare most of the recipes in this book on the spur of the moment. (You probably have some of them on hand already.) If you feel like expanding your repertoire, you can branch out with other suggested foods as the spirit or a specific recipe moves you.

Almost all of the ingredients used in this book are available at supermarkets and natural food stores, with an occasional foray into a specialty or Asian grocery. During the course of my travels and while testing recipes for this book, I have experimented with numerous brands and developed preferences. For a complete glossary of ingredients including recommended brands, see Ingredients at a Glance (page 148).

ten strategies for short-cut cooking

1. *Build* flavor fast by using "secret" ingredients that provide intense taste by the spoonful.

2. *Be creative* with carefully selected high-quality instant and prepared foods.

3. *Explore* the versatility of organic canned staples such as beans and diced tomatoes.

4. *Prepare* the whole meal in one pot whenever possible. While the longer-cooking ingredients are simmering away, prepare the items to be added toward the end.

5. *Cook* in quantity and freeze extra for later use.

6. *Develop* an imaginative repertoire of quick-cooking dishes using fresh ingredients that are easy to keep on hand because they don't spoil quickly—for example, cabbage, potatoes, and carrots.

7. *Become acquainted* with quick-cooking grains like polenta, quinoa, and couscous. Set a kettle of water over high heat even before you take the grains out of the cupboard.

8. *Rely* on the tool or appliance that will get the job done most efficiently.

9. *Make* a mix for "fun food" like scones, waffles, and cookies—and freeze it in batches for quick treats down the road.

10. *Don't take cooking (or life) too seriously!*

at room temperature

the basics

miscellaneous cans and jars

chickpeas, navy or cannellini beans, and black beans

diced tomatoes with green chilies

diced or crushed tomatoes

tomato-based pasta sauce and salsa

roasted red peppers

pasta and grains

various shapes and sizes, such as tiny (orzo or tubettini), medium (orrecchiette or shells), and long (spaghetti or fettuccine)

white rice (basmati or jasmine and extra-long-grain)

instant polenta

fresh vegetables

garlic, onions, potatoes, and winter squash

branching out

miscellaneous cans and jars

pinto beans, lentils, red kidney beans, and black soybeans

chinese vegetables, such as bamboo shoots, baby corn, straw mushrooms, and water chestnuts

coconut milk

pasta and grains

asian-style noodles, such as brown-rice udon, soba, or rice noodles

quick-cooking barley

fresh vegetables

plum or beefsteak tomatoes, avocados

miscellaneous

dried beans, such as black, navy, and chickpeas

instant black and refried beans

sun-dried tomatoes (oil-packed)

arame and instant wakame flakes

silken tofu (in aseptic package)

baking soda and baking powder

in the freezer

You might be surprised to find grains, nuts, and flours on this list, but these items will keep longer in the freezer than at room temperature.

the basics

frozen vegetables

corn, chopped spinach, and peas

uncooked grains

whole wheat couscous, brown rice, and quinoa

home-cooked brown rice (see page 43)

branching out

miscellaneous

home-cooked beans in 1¾-cup portions (see page 28)

frozen lima beans and artichoke hearts

unsweetened, grated, dried coconut

nuts, such as walnuts and almonds, and seeds, such as sesame and sunflower

whole-grain pastry and all-purpose white flours

in the refrigerator

the basics

`fresh vegetables`

cabbage, carrots, and scallions

`miscellaneous`

fresh parsley and cilantro

lemons

roasted garlic and basil olive oil, plain olive oil, toasted sesame oil

note: The oils may solidify in the refrigerator but will liquefy when brought to room temperature. If you're in a hurry, hold the bottle under hot running water or remove the cap and pop it into the microwave for ten to fifteen seconds.

branching out

`fresh vegetables`

spinach, chard, kale, leeks, jalapeños, red bell peppers, portobello mushrooms, celery

`miscellaneous`

fresh basil, dill, mint, and ginger

quick-toasting nuts and seeds

Pop nuts or seeds into a toaster oven on its tray or in a shallow pan and toast them at 350 degrees until fragrant and slightly darkened, 3 to 4 minutes. Or, toast seeds in a nonstick skillet over medium-high heat, stirring constantly.

storing fresh herbs

To keep more delicate leafy fresh herbs (such as parsley, dill, and cilantro) for about a week in the refrigerator, submerge about two inches of the roots and stems in a glass of water and cover the leaves with a plastic bag. The flavor diminishes slightly over time.

Herbs with woody stems and small leaves (such as rosemary and oregano) may be refrigerated in perforated plastic vegetable bags and will last about ten days.

saffron (I always refrigerate saffron to preserve its fragrance)

limes

fresh tofu

rosemary olive oil and hot pepper sesame oil

black oil-cured and green pimento-stuffed olives

pure maple syrup

condiments and seasonings

the basics

miscellaneous

sea salt

instant vegetable stock powder

salt

Salt is so basic to our cooking vocabulary that it's easy to forget that not all salt is created equal. I once did a blind tasting of various salts and was amazed to discover that some had a harsh edge while others delivered subtle sweetness or pleasing citric overtones.

I prefer to cook with a high-quality sea salt, which has a mellow taste and contains trace minerals. In addition, it is free of the additives (such as dextrose, calcium silicate, and potassium iodide) commonly found in supermarket brands of salt.

For day-to-day cooking, I use Lima sea salt, available in natural food stores. For delicate preparations where a slight citric edge would enhance flavor, I use a light-gray Breton sea salt, which is expensive but absolutely delicious. You can find it in some gourmet shops or mail-order it from Goldmine (see Mail-Order Sources).

dijon mustard

tomato paste

balsamic vinegar

tamari and/or shoyu

dried herbs and spices

italian herb blend (page 16 or store-bought)

mild curry blend (page 17 or store-bought)

chili powder

crushed red pepper flakes

cumin seeds

black peppercorns

branching out

dried herbs and spices

herbes de provence (page 17 or store-bought)

black (brown) mustard seeds

chipotle chili powder (see page 150)

rosemary and oregano

coriander seeds

ground cinnamon

miscellaneous

brown rice and sherry wine vinegars

liquid smoke

storing and freezing leftover canned tomato paste

Freeze leftovers in one-tablespoon amounts on a baking sheet lined with waxed paper. Once they're frozen, transfer the spoonfuls to a Ziploc freezer bag. Add the amount you need directly to a pot of hot liquid and it will quickly defrost. (Yes, I find tomato paste in a tube very convenient, but the canned variety is much more economical.)

storing and grinding spices

Store all spices (and dried herbs) away from heat and light, preferably in glass bottles. If possible, buy them in small quantities (about one ounce) and replenish at least every six months (after that, their flavors begin to fade off into oblivion).

For optimum taste, grind whole spices as needed in a mini-chopper or coffee grinder set aside for this purpose. Cinnamon sticks are one exception, since they can be tricky to grind; buying already ground cinnamon is a more convenient and very acceptable option.

a short primer on veggie (and tofu) prep

You don't have to be a Japanese sushi chef to chop efficiently. With a sharp knife or a food processor and a willingness to dispense with perfectionism, you too can coarsely chop an onion or shred cabbage in a minute or two. Here are some tips, in alphabetical order by ingredient, on preparing the vegetables used in this book.

shredding cabbage: Remove any bruised or limp outside leaves. Quarter the cabbage and slice away the hard central core. Slice each quarter very thin with a serrated knife, or use the shredding disk of your food processor.

chopping carrots: Trim and scrub (if organic) or peel. Cut each into four chunks, place in a food processor fitted with the metal blade, and pulse until chopped to the desired size. Scrape down the bowl once or twice if necessary.

mincing garlic: To minimize peeling time, select heads of garlic that have large cloves. For easier peeling, lay the wide part of a chef's knife on each clove and bang down on it with the heel of your hand. Or, you can purchase an inexpensive small rubber tube called E-Z-Rol, which quickly separates the skin from individual cloves. Cut the peeled clove(s) in half and process in a mini-chopper, or mince by hand. If a recipe also calls for chopped onion, you can use the pulsing action of a food processor to chop the onion and garlic together.

grating ginger: Trim, then peel (or just rinse if the skin is thin). Rub one end against a fine grater or, if the ginger is young and not fibrous, cut into small pieces and mince in a mini-chopper. Or, toss small pieces through the feed tube of the food processor while the motor is running.

removing fresh herb leaves from the stems: For leafy herbs, such as parsley and cilantro, hold the bunch together and cut off the leaves just at the point where most of the leaves meet the stems. When chopping, include the bits of stem still attached to leaves. (Only mature large basil leaves need to be picked from their stems one by one.)

For herbs with woody stems, such as rosemary and thyme, hold each sprig at the top. Run your fingers down the stem, and the leaves will come off in small clumps that can be chopped if necessary.

seeding fresh chilies: Trim off the stem end of the chile and slice it in half lengthwise. Scoop out the seeds and veins with a teaspoon and discard. To avoid skin irritation, wear rubber gloves when handling chilies, or wash your hands well after you are finished.

getting the sand out of leeks: Trim off the root end and remove any bruised or yellowed outer leaves. Thinly slice the white and light green parts into thin rounds. Push through the centers of the rounds to separate into rings. Swish vigorously in a large bowl of water, and lift out with a slotted spoon. Repeat in fresh water if necessary. Transfer to a colander and rinse thoroughly.

reconstituting and cleaning dried mushrooms: Steep the dried mushrooms in boiling water in a covered bowl or pot until soft, about 15 minutes. Lift them out with a slotted spoon, leaving any sand behind. Rinse the mushrooms carefully, and cut away any gritty sections. Strain the soaking liquid through moistened cheesecloth or a wet clean paper coffee filter and use as part of the liquid called for in your recipe.

chopping onions: Peel the onions. To coarsely chop: Trim off the root and top of each onion and cut lengthwise in half. Set cut side down and thinly slice the onion lengthwise. Holding the slices together, give the onion a quarter turn and thinly slice crosswise. To finely chop onions, use a food processor: Quarter them and place in the work bowl fitted with the metal blade. Pulse five or six times, scraping down the bowl once or twice, until the onions are finely chopped. Never let the food processor run at full steam, or the onions will turn to mush.

roasting red peppers: To use a gas stove, place one pepper per burner on the gas burner grid. Turn the flame to high and roast until the pepper is completely blackened and charred on the underside. Give the pepper a quarter turn with a pair of long tongs (avoid forks or skewers, which would pierce the pepper and release the juices), and continue to roast and turn until the pepper is charred all around. Or, roast the peppers

storing fresh tofu

For the most convenient and healthful option, purchase organic fresh tofu sold in one-pound plastic tubs in the refrigerator section of health food stores. Unopened, the tofu will remain fresh until at least the expiration date. Once it's opened, submerge any leftover tofu in fresh water in a tightly sealed container and refrigerate. Change the water daily, and the tofu will last for about one week.

To extend storage time, drain and freeze the tofu in a well-sealed container for up to three months. Defrost before using, then squeeze out excess water by gently pressing the block between two plates tipped over the sink. Slice as directed in the recipe. Tofu that has been frozen darkens slightly, develops a chewy texture, and absorbs sauce like a sponge.

under a preheated gas or electric broiler, turning as needed. (This is one case where you don't have to worry about burning, so feel free to do other tasks in between turns.)

Place the charred peppers in a brown paper or plastic bag, fold over the top, and let steam for 15 minutes. Rub off the charred skin, rinsing your hands frequently as you go. Cut the peppers in half and remove the seeds and ribs. If not using immediately, cut into strips, place in a sealed container, cover with a thin layer of olive oil, and refrigerate for up to one week.

trimming snow peas: Snap off the stem end and gently pull to remove the "string" from the seam(s) of the pod.

peeling butternut squash: Cut the squash lengthwise in half and scoop out the seeds. Set it cut side down on the counter and peel each half before cutting into chunks or dice; for finer chopping, pulse chunks in a food processor fitted with the steel blade.

washing spinach: Discard any bruised or discolored leaves. Swish vigorously in a large bowl (or shallow sinkful) of water. Transfer the spinach to a colander. Empty the bowl (or sink), rinse it thoroughly, and refill with fresh water. Repeat the process until the spinach is completely free of sand.

dicing a one-pound block of tofu: Drain the tofu and set it on a small chopping board with a long side facing you. Using a serrated knife, gently cut into ½-inch horizontal slices. Holding the block together, cut crosswise into ½-inch slices. Give the chopping board a quarter turn and cut into ½-inch slices to create dice.

essential tools and equipment

A limited number of carefully selected appliances, tools, and cookware can make noteworthy reductions in food preparation and cooking times. Although I find it quite relaxing to chop vegetables by hand, there are occasions when it's much more practical to team up with my Cuisinart and get the job done quickly.

basic appliances and tools

I'm not a big fan of small electrics, but there are a few "plug-ins" that I wouldn't be without.

I consider a food processor essential for chopping large quantities of vegetables, shredding cabbage, blending dressings, and pureeing soups. (Although a blender does a better job of the latter, I rarely bother to take it down from the shelf.) I keep my Cuisinart Pro 14 permanently stationed on my countertop and have recently replaced that newfangled click-in lid, which I hated from day one, with the old-fashioned type of lid that came with the original processors. (I was surprised to learn that it is still available and am mentioning it in case you are interested; however, the feed tube is smaller).

I almost always use my mini-chopper to mince garlic and ginger. Unfortunately the inexpensive SEP model I own and love is no longer available (but see the information on immersion blenders below). I reserve a coffee grinder specifically for grinding spices; I have always found the bottom-of-the-line Krups models reliable.

My favorite vegetable peeler is one made by Kuhn-Rikon (available through Williams-Sonoma and Zabar's), because it is well designed, feels good in the hand, and stays sharp for a long time. The Good Grips peeler is also terrific and more readily available.

There are no substitutes for a high-quality chef's knife, a steel for keeping it sharp, and a chopping block to go with it! A long serrated knife is very useful for slicing bread, cabbage, and tomatoes.

I find a small pair of kitchen scissors indispensable for opening packages and snipping fresh herbs.

branching out: An immersion blender can puree soups and sauces right in the pot, saving time and cleanup. It is a relative newcomer to my kitchen, but I find myself using it more and more. The Braun model comes with a useful mini-chopper attachment that's great for mincing herbs and garlic.

essentials for cooking

I bought a microwave oven when I began working on this book, and I expected to hate it. But, like many other cooks, I've come to depend on it for quick defrosting and reheating—really impressive for grains. And it cooks certain vegetables beautifully too. (You'll learn my favorites in the vegetable chapter.)

A large nonstick saucepan can be a virtual workhorse in the kitchen. I'm very happy with my four-quart Farberware Millennium, which has a long-lasting nonstick surface and a well-constructed bottom that cooks evenly and discourages scorching.

I don't understand how people can live without a toaster oven. Not only do I use it daily for my morning toast (no bread ever gets stuck in it!), but it's also handy for toasting nuts, baking one or two potatoes, and reheating scones and waffles. Because it is so small, a toaster oven reaches the desired temperature almost instantly.

branching out: I am probably America's number one (and most vocal) pressure cooker fan. Pressure cookers are unbeatable for turning out a nine-minute lentil soup, cooking chickpeas in sixteen minutes, and making risotto in five minutes—without stirring. You will find a few recipes in this book adapted to this wondrous appliance. The new models imported from Europe are 100 percent safe.

For stir-frying vegetables, I recommend the stainless steel chef's pan (with lid) by All-Clad rather than an ordinary wok. It is easier to clean than the less-expensive carbon steel woks and has a flat bottom so you don't have to fuss with a stand. All-Clad's twelve-inch nonstick frying pan (with lid) is also excellent for stir-frying.

the building blocks of short-cut vegetarian cooking

After years of searching for short-cuts in my vegetarian kitchen, I've discovered that my most successful recipes involve one or more of the following strategies:

build flavor fast with a select group of ingredients, such as high-quality instant vegetable stock powder, seasoning blends, and infused olive oils—ingredients that add complex flavor by the spoonful.

make homemade and carefully selected store-bought sauces an integral part of cooking to create memorable dips, spreads, salads, and stir-fries.

use quick-cooking or precooked ingredients that are uncompromising, such as instant polenta, whole wheat couscous, and canned organic or frozen home-cooked beans as the basis for a number of delicious dishes.

use the tool or appliance that will get the job done most efficiently. In this chapter, I'll go into the first three strategies in some depth. You'll get a clear idea of my fourth strategy by glancing at pages 11–12 in the preceding chapter and by cooking your way through the recipes.

instant vegetable stock powder

Instant vegetable stock powder is a major player in my recipes because it contributes the flavors of a dozen or so herbs and vegetables without any shopping, cleaning, or chopping!

I used to feel embarrassed about using stock powder instead of homemade vegetable stock, but the day I realized that my risotto actually tasted better when I used my favorite stock powder instead of homemade stock, I decided to come forward with my preference. Although it's not impossible, it's time-consuming (and expensive) to make the kind of intensely flavored vegetable stock that a few teaspoons of high-quality powder can deliver.

Once I did a blind testing of about ten different brands of instant vegetable stock and was shocked at the fluctuations in quality and flavor. Some brands were unpalatably bitter, others horribly salty. Indeed, the brand that I'd been using regularly ended up being one of my least favorites.

Vogue Instant Vege Base ranked highest in the tasting, based on its excellent flavor. Sure enough, the label revealed the product to be an organic, low-sodium, preservative-free blend of soybeans, dehydrated vegetables, herbs, and brewer's yeast. I used it exclusively to test the recipes in this book; however, my testers reported fine results using a few other brands. (To order Vege Base directly or to find a local distributor, call Vogue at 305–458–2915.)

If you can't find Vogue Vege Base, look for a Swiss brand called Morga, or the Frontier-brand vegetable stock powder that many natural food stores sell in bulk. Failing these, I suggest doing your own blind tasting using the brands that are available in your area. (By the way, I don't recommend using canned vegetable broth. It is not at all economical or practical—who wants to drag home all that liquid?—and those I've tasted don't match the best instant stocks for flavor or quality.)

Obviously, instant stock makes a great base for quick soups, but the taste of stews and pilafs also deepens if you stir in a teaspoon or two. To increase intensity, I often add the stock powder more generously than the one teaspoon (or one cube) per cup of water that most package instructions suggest. However, increasing the proportion of stock powder must be done judiciously to keep its flavor in the background.

One precaution: Since the amount of salt in instant stocks varies widely, in recipes that use stock powder, I have deliberately called for less salt than I normally add and suggested that adjustments be made before serving.

seasoning blends

For the hurry-up cook, using a tried-and-true premixed blend of herbs or spices is a guaranteed way to achieve great taste without waiting for the herbal muse to appear.

Two of the seasoning mixtures I use frequently with great success are homemade Italian Herb Blend and Mild Curry Powder. For additional variety, I keep a classic Herbes de Provence on hand. This blend provides a good alternative for Mediterranean-inspired dishes, but the first two are more versatile and have become my old reliables.

All three blends can be purchased at a supermarket or specialty food shop, but it's worth the few extra minutes to make your own—particularly curry powder, which varies dramatically from one brand to the next and quickly loses freshness. (I do, however, have a few reliable brands to recommend; see Ingredients at a Glance.)

Consider these seasoning blend recipes as guidelines and increase or decrease ingredients to suit your own personal taste. If you find yourself using up the blends quickly, make double batches—but keep in mind that dried herbs and ground spices lose intensity over time.

italian herb blend

prep: 5 minutes

1 tablespoon dried oregano

1 tablespoon dried basil

2 teaspoons dried thyme

2 teaspoons dried rosemary

1 ½ teaspoons fennel seeds

1 teaspoon crushed red pepper flakes (optional)

Combine all of the herbs in a small wide-mouthed jar. Shake well. Store in a dark, cool place for up to 3 months.

makes about ¼ cup

Some combination of Italian herbs is on every supermarket spice shelf, but I've arrived at a formula I love. If you do opt for a supermarket brand, add some fennel seeds for an inspired touch. My recipe calls for dried herb leaves rather than ground herbs; the latter lose their vibrancy quickly and taste like sawdust.

mild curry blend

2 tablespoons coriander seeds

1 tablespoon cumin seeds

2 teaspoons black (brown) mustard seeds

1 teaspoon fennel seeds

½ tablespoon ground turmeric

¼ teaspoon ground cinnamon

⅛ teaspoon cayenne

prep: under 10 minutes

Place the coriander, cumin, mustard, and fennel seeds in a spice grinder and grind to a fine powder. Transfer to a small wide-mouthed jar and stir in the remaining spices. Cover and refrigerate for up to 2 months.

makes about ¼ cup

Every Indian cook has a favorite curry blend. Many classic recipes call for toasting the spices before grinding them, but I prefer using them as is.

This curry blend is quite mild but can be made hotter by adding more cayenne. Keep it refrigerated to maintain optimum flavor.

herbes de provence

1 tablespoon dried basil

2 teaspoons dried tarragon

2 teaspoons dried summer savory

2 teaspoons dried rosemary

2 teaspoons dried marjoram

2 teaspoons dried chervil (optional)

prep: 5 minutes

This combination of herbs is a pleasant alternative to the Italian seasoning blend, offering a simple way to put a "new face" on many recipes in this book. Substitute it in an equal amount. Some French cooks add dried

This combination of herbs is a pleasant alternative to the Italian seasoning blend, offering a simple way to put a "new face" on many recipes in this book. Substitute it in an equal amount. Some French cooks add dried lavender to their Provençal mix, but I'd rather smell lavender than taste it in my soup. Be sure to use whole leaves, not ground herbs.

homemade infused oils?

Although it's easy to make herb-infused oils at home, it's not practical for the short-cut cook because they easily develop mold and must therefore be made in small quantities and used quickly. However, I've included some basic instructions here for those who don't have a local source of infused oils.

Warm ½ cup olive oil in a small saucepan over low heat with 3 tablespoons chopped fresh basil or rosemary. Remove from the heat and let steep for 1 hour; strain. Refrigerate and use within 1 week.

As for roasted garlic oil, I prefer the hassle-free bottled variety; homemade versions are more complicated to make and don't always taste as good.

lavender to their Provençal mix, but I'd rather smell lavender than taste it in my soup. Be sure to use whole leaves, not ground herbs.

Combine all of the herbs in a small wide-mouthed jar. Shake well. Store in a dark, cool place for up to 3 months.

makes about ¼ cup

infused oils

I am a passionate user of the infused oils made popular in recent years. Indeed, I consider my refrigerator empty if there are no roasted garlic and basil oils on hand. High-quality infused oils need be used very sparingly. Even a teaspoon or two will add dimension to any dish—particularly when stirred in just before serving.

Infused oils shrink preparation time. When you use roasted garlic oil, you needn't peel and mince garlic cloves—plus you get the roasted garlic's warm, mellow taste.

Paired with balsamic vinegar or lemon juice, infused oils make excellent splash-on dressings for salads and pasta. You can also use them to whip up a batch of my Very Versatile Vinaigrette (page 19).

Although I use the roasted (not raw!) garlic and basil oils most frequently, I like to have the more pungent rosemary oil on hand as well. I like these three flavors in the Consorzio line. (I don't find the other flavors—such as oregano, porcini, or five-pepper—as versatile.) Consorzio and two other reliable brands, Loriva and Boyajian, are widely distributed through gourmet and cookware shops, and in many upscale supermarkets.

Once they've been opened, it's best to store oils in the refrigerator, where they will last for many months. Since some of them solidify, remember to remove the ones you need from the fridge "to thaw" about half an hour before you begin to cook. If you forget, run the bottle under hot water for a few minutes to "melt" the solidified oil, or pop the bottle (remove the cap if it is metal) into the microwave for 15 seconds.

very versatile vinaigrette

¼ cup basil olive oil

2 tablespoons roasted garlic olive oil

4 to 5 tablespoons Cavalli balsamic vinegar
   (start with 3 tablespoons if using another brand)

¾ teaspoon Dijon mustard

¾ teaspoon salt, or more to taste

Freshly ground black pepper to taste (optional)

prep: 5 minutes

In a jar, mix the oils with ¼ cup vinegar, the mustard, salt, and pepper (if using). Shake well. Add more vinegar and salt to taste if necessary, keeping in mind that the potency of the dressing will be diluted once it is tossed with a salad. Refrigerate until about a half hour before needed. Shake vigorously before using.

makes about ½ cup

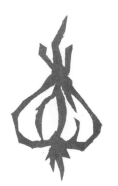

This is an elegant, memorable vinaigrette, created from two different infused oils and a high-quality balsamic vinegar. The recipe reflects my preference for a roughly equal balance of oil and acid. The sweetness of the balsamic vinegar is balanced by a bit of Dijon mustard. Freshly squeezed lemon juice makes a fine alternative to the vinegar, but only if you plan to use the vinaigrette within a few days.

The vinaigrette lasts for a couple of months under refrigeration, so you can double or triple the recipe. Try brushing it onto vegetables headed for the grill or roasting pan. It also adds a touch of class to mesclun as well as to pasta, bean, and grain salads. If using the vinaigrette on bean or grain salads, you're likely to need a bit more vinegar or lemon juice once the salad has been tossed.

saucy solutions

Go to a natural food store that maintains high selection standards, and you'll see a mind-boggling array of prepared sauces, salsas, and salad dressings—all free of the preservatives and other artificial ingredients that are typically found in their supermarket look-alikes.

Unfortunately, not all products sold in health food stores are created equal, and some taste much better than others. To help you avoid disappointments, I've recommended some favorite brands in Ingredients at a Glance, page 148. As a general rule, I opt for organic salsa and spaghetti sauce, and I also splurge on a particular salad dressing that I can't figure out how to reproduce at home.

However, because it is costly to buy bottled sauces and dressings, I've developed a small repertoire of splash-on vinaigrettes, stir-fry sauces, and mustard-based enhancements for steamed vegetables. Some are so quick to prepare that I make them on the spot. Others—like the two stir-fry sauces (pages 25 and 26) or Lemon-Tahini Sauce (page 23)—take a few minutes to pull together, so I usually make about a cupful at a time, refrigerate whatever's left, and replace as needed.

Both homemade and store-bought sauces offer a variety of uses beyond the obvious. For example, pasta sauce added to soups and stews provides body and multiple levels of flavor, as you can see in the recipe for Pasta Fagioli with Cabbage on page 93. And there's more to salsa than a dip for chips. Straight from the bottle, a good salsa can become the basis for a terrific fast chili or ready-made sauce for a southwestern potato salad (see recipes on pages 86 and 79).

A delicious salad dressing can turn thinly sliced cabbage into an unusual instant slaw. For this purpose, I usually turn to the outrageously good Annie's Shiitake & Sesame Vinaigrette. I also drizzle this dressing on steamed and stir-fried vegetables, boiled grains, and baked potatoes.

mustard sauces

When I'm thinking "quick sauce," my mind frequently turns to Dijon mustard, because it supplies both heat and depth of flavor. As a result, you'll find numerous mustard-based sauces scattered throughout this book: a garlicky mustard sauce on page 95, a maple-tamari version below, and a stir-fry sauce on page 26.

Once you've found a favorite mustard-based sauce, you'll no doubt think of many ways to use it—mashed into baked potatoes, drizzled onto steamed vegetables, or tossed with bean and grain salads.

I favor Maille, an excellent brand of mustard made in Dijon by traditional methods, but you can try these recipes with the mustard of your choice.

lemony maple-mustard dressing

¼ cup tamari

prep: 5 minutes

2 tablespoons Dijon mustard

2 tablespoons pure maple syrup

2 to 4 tablespoons freshly squeezed lemon juice

This is a great fat-free dressing for bean and grain salads. Try especially the Pinto Bean Salad on page 77—a personal favorite.

In a wide-mouthed jar, combine the tamari, mustard, maple syrup, and 2 tablespoons lemon juice. Shake well. Taste and add enough additional lemon juice to give the sauce a distinct puckery edge. Refrigerate for up to 1 week.

note: Leftovers will need to be perked up with additional fresh lemon juice, and sometimes you'll need to add more lemon juice once you've tossed the dressing with salad ingredients.

makes about ½ cup

sauces from nuts and seeds

Once found only in ethnic markets, spicy Asian peanut sauces and mellow sesame tahini have found a place in many American kitchens. With their creamy texture and intense flavor, nut butters make ideal bases for delicious sauces that require few additional ingredients. Double or triple these recipes and explore their versatility in a variety of green, grain, and bean dishes.

Store leftover sauce in the refrigerator, where it will thicken considerably. To thin, stir in a tablespoon (or slightly more) of hot water or pop into the microwave for 10 to 20 seconds.

asian peanut sauce

I cup unsalted nonhydrogenated peanut butter

2½ tablespoons tamari or shoyu

I to 2 teaspoons brown rice or seasoned rice vinegar

¼ to ½ teaspoon cayenne (depending upon your tolerance for heat)

⅔ to ¾ cup boiling water

Finely minced garlic and fresh ginger to taste (optional)

prep: 5 minutes

Place the peanut butter, tamari, rice vinegar, cayenne, and ⅔ cup boiling water in the bowl of a food processor. Process to blend, adding additional boiling water if necessary to create a thick but pourable sauce. Use immediately, or transfer to a jar and refrigerate for up to 2 weeks. When ready to serve, blend in garlic and ginger to the portion you'll be using. If necessary, thin the sauce to the desired consistency with hot water.

makes about 1½ cups

With this sauce on hand, you can create a multitude of habit-forming dishes. Toss peanut sauce with pasta and grains as well as steamed vegetables, salads, and slaws. When chilled, it's thick enough to use as a condiment on a sandwich of grilled vegetables.

There's less tamari here than I use at home. Add more if you like once the dressing is tossed with the other ingredients.

lemon-tahini sauce

Small bunch (about 30 sprigs) flat-leaf parsley

prep: about 10 minutes

½ cup sesame tahini

2 to 4 large cloves garlic

4 to 5 tablespoons freshly squeezed lemon juice

2 to 6 tablespoons water

¾ teaspoon salt, or to taste

⅛ teaspoon cayenne (optional)

Holding the parsley in a bunch, trim off and discard an inch or so from the bottom of the stems. Cut the bunch crosswise into thirds. Place in a colander, rinse, and drain. Bounce the colander up and down to shake off excess water.

Place the tahini, parsley, garlic, 4 tablespoons lemon juice, and 2 tablespoons water into the bowl of a food processor. Blend well, scraping down the sides of the bowl as needed and adding enough additional water and/or lemon juice to create a sauce with a smooth, pourable consistency and a nice puckery taste. (The amount of liquid you'll need to add will depend upon the thickness of the tahini and how much water adhered to the parsley.) Add the salt and cayenne (if using). Refrigerate until needed, for up to 1 week.

makes about 1 cup

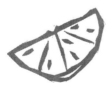

When I tasted this sauce in Jerusalem a few years ago, I was reminded of how much I like the earthy taste of sesame tahini and the brightness of parsley —stems and all.

Whip up a batch and toss it with grains and chopped carrots for a colorful salad (see page 72), blend it with cooked chickpeas for a quick sandwich filling (see page 50), or spoon it over microwaved kale or steamed broccoli florets set on a bed of brown rice for an entrée.

The amount of garlic you'll need depends upon your taste. I like to start with two cloves and blend in more if needed —keeping in mind that the sauce's flavor will be somewhat diluted when mixed with other ingredients.

Refrigerate for up to one week. Thin as needed with additional fresh lemon juice —or water, if you're out of lemons.

two stir-fry sauces

I felt impelled to develop a homemade stir-fry sauce after purchasing a few store-bought versions that were expensive and disappointing. (If you have a favorite brand, feel free to use it whenever a recipe in this book calls for a stir-fry sauce.)

I created the luscious Sesame-Ginger Stir-Fry Sauce (page 25) first, but realized that it would be nice to have an option for those who are carefully monitoring fat grams. Mustard once again came to the rescue in a low-fat, flavor-packed Maple and Mustard Stir-Fry Sauce (page 26).

These sauces can turn a variety of chopped and canned Asian vegetables into stir-fried meals on short notice. The recipes on pages 97–100 will give you some good ideas and can be used as prototypes for your own creations. If you find yourself going through either of the sauces all too quickly, just double the recipe the next time you make it.

sesame-ginger stir-fry sauce

2 tablespoons sesame seeds

¼ cup roasted garlic olive oil or peanut oil

2 tablespoons toasted sesame oil

3 tablespoons tamari or shoyu

¼ to ⅓ cup Japanese-style pickled ginger

2 tablespoons pickled ginger juice (drained from the pickled ginger; see Note)

2 tablespoons boiling water

prep: about 10 minutes

Place the sesame seeds in a shallow baking dish or other ovenproof container. (I use an aluminum one recycled from take-out food.) Toast in a toaster oven at 375 degrees until fragrant, 2 to 3 minutes. (Or, toast in a non-stick skillet over medium-high heat, stirring constantly.) Transfer to a plate and let cool.

In a food processor or blender, combine all of the ingredients except the water and toasted sesame seeds. With the motor running, add the boiling water and process until the sauce is thoroughly blended. Transfer the sauce to a glass jar and add the sesame seeds. Cover and refrigerate until needed, up to 3 months. Shake vigorously before using.

note: If you don't have enough pickled ginger juice, substitute brown-rice vinegar or seasoned rice vinegar to taste.

makes about ¾ cup

This recipe may send you chasing around a bit for ingredients, but the taste rewards effort. I've chosen to use pickled ginger and roasted garlic olive oil so that you can refrigerate this homemade sauce for up to three months. (Fresh ginger and garlic would considerably reduce storage time.)

If you choose to use peanut rather than roasted garlic olive oil, you can mince a clove or two of garlic to add to individual stir-fry recipes. Use the larger amount of pickled ginger if you love the flavor and want it to predominate.

This is a convenient alternative to the preceding recipe, as I suspect that most of the ingredients are already in your refrigerator. Despite the limited number of ingredients, it is exceedingly tasty.

Because this sauce is lower in fat than the sesame-ginger sauce, you may need to add an extra tablespoon or two more than suggested in the recipes calling for stir-fry sauce.

maple and mustard stir-fry sauce

¼ cup tamari or shoyu

¼ cup Dijon mustard

3 tablespoons water

3 tablespoons toasted sesame oil

2 tablespoons pure maple syrup

prep: about 5 minutes

In a jar, combine all of the ingredients. Cover and shake vigorously. Refrigerate until needed, up to 3 months. Shake well before using.

makes about ¾ cup

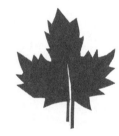

the salsa spirit

The extraordinary popularity of salsa makes you wish you'd bought stock in one of the better-known companies. In addition to all of its other tasty virtues, salsa can become the short-cut cook's secret weapon, contributing vibrancy and complexity to otherwise simple dishes.

I've never gotten into the habit of making homemade salsa, perhaps because I live in New York City, where terrific tomatoes are few and far between. In addition, I find many brands of store-bought salsa very appealing and hard to beat.

Make the effort to find a salsa whose balance of flavors and spiciness excites your palate. Because the success of recipes using salsa depends so heavily on its flavor, a brand that is too acidic, garlicky, or hot can result in disaster.

To avoid such disappointment, keep experimenting or ask your friends to recommend their favorites until you find a brand (or brands) that you really like. Some dependable, inexpensive, and readily available bottled choices are Enrico's and Newman's Own. If you're fond of smoky flavors, for a delicious splurge, try Timpone's Salsa Muy Rica or El Paso Chile Company's Chipotle Cha Cha Cha. (These latter two are especially delightful in the Southwest Potato Salad, on page 79, and Smoky Black Bean Chili, on page 86.) And you may be lucky enough to find local fresh salsas that are really outstanding.

At the risk of getting boos from cooks devoted to banning every last gram of fat from their diets, I must admit that I find some fat-free salsas (and pasta sauces) too acidic. If you do too, a good solution is to stir just a tablespoon or two of olive oil into the jar; this way you are controlling your fat intake but creating a better balance of flavors.

Unless it is otherwise specified, when preparing recipes that call for salsa, use a tomato-based version that is not studded with beans or corn.

full of beans

Having an inventory of home-cooked beans gives you a major head start in getting a healthy dinner on the table quickly. Although I always have a good selection of organic canned beans on my shelves, there's no question that cooking your own beans is more economical and offers a much larger variety to choose from—including lovely scarlet runners, Christmas limas, and black lentils, to name but a few. Because of their flavor, sturdiness, and versatility, the three varieties I use most often are chickpeas, navy beans, and black (turtle) beans. They all make good candidates for this home-inventory approach.

When preparing beans from scratch, a good short-cut is to make much more than you need. Cook 1 pound (about 2½ cups) of dried beans at a time. This amount will yield 5 to 6 cups after cooking. Drain the cooked beans thoroughly. Once they are completely cooled, divide them among three Ziploc freezer bags (about 1¾ cups per bag). Refrigerate the beans you plan to use over the next few days. Label, date, and freeze the remaining bags and use them within 3 months.

For those times when you don't have home-cooked beans on hand, organic canned beans are the best alternative. Look for a low-sodium brand and you won't even have to rinse them. In fact, you can use the flavorful cooking liquid in your dish (or substitute it for some of the vegetable stock called for in soup recipes).

Happily, the variety of canned organic beans keeps expanding. Most recently, black soybeans, lentils, and a range of seasoned beans (such as chili and barbecued) have become available. Canned beans are particularly useful when making bean salads, which require specimens that are fully cooked yet still firm and shapely—a state that it takes practice (and luck!) to achieve when cooking beans from scratch at home.

My own personal philosophy is to eat as much organic food as possible. Although the price of organic canned beans is becoming more competitive, you may still choose to opt for less-expensive supermarket brands. In that case, be sure to discard the canning liquid and rinse the beans thoroughly to wash away excessive saltiness.

All of the recipes in this book call for 1¾ cups of beans—the approximate amount contained in a 15-ounce can—so that you can use either home-cooked or purchased beans.

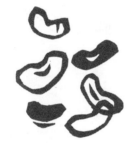

beans under pressure

Use approximately 3 cups of water for each cup of beans. **Do not fill the cooker more than halfway.**

Add 2 teaspoons of oil for every cup of beans. The oil prevents foaming, which might catapult a bean skin into the vent. If you like, add a large onion, quartered, a few garlic cloves, and 2 large bay leaves. Lock the lid into place and bring up to high pressure.

for large (soaked) beans, such as chickpeas or scarlet runners: Cook for 10 minutes under pressure, then allow the pressure to come down naturally.

for medium (soaked) beans, such as pintos or black beans: Cook for 3 minutes under pressure, then allow the pressure to come down naturally.

for small (soaked) beans, such as navy beans or adukis: Cook for 2 minutes under pressure, then allow the pressure to come down naturally.

Test the beans for doneness. If more cooking is required, set the lid slightly ajar and simmer until done.

Drain the beans. Remove and discard the onion, garlic, and bay leaves if you used them. Let cool completely before dividing into portion sizes as described on page 28.

presoaking beans

Even when pressure-cooking beans, I prefer to presoak them in ample water to cover for at least four hours, or overnight, then drain off the soaking water. This extra step results in greater digestibility and more even cooking. If you haven't planned in advance and presoaked the beans, you can try this pressure cooker speed-soak technique.

Bring the beans up to high pressure in ample water to cover.

for large beans: Cook for 2 minutes under pressure and allow the pressure to come down naturally.

for medium beans: Cook for 1 minute under pressure and allow the pressure to come down naturally.

for small beans: As soon as high pressure is reached, turn off the heat, and allow the pressure to come down naturally.

Drain the beans and cook them under pressure or by the standard stove-top method.

note: If you don't have time to cook the beans after they've soaked, you can drain and refrigerate them for up to 2 days or freeze them for up to 2 months. Defrost them before cooking. Soaked beans that have been frozen take about 10 percent less time to cook, but they don't hold their shape as well.

the pressure come down naturally minimizes damage to the beans' skins. If the beans are not tender by the time all the pressure has been released, simmer them until done with the lid ajar, keeping a watchful eye to avoid overcooking.

If time permits, it's best to soak the beans first. For instructions, see page 30.

cooking beans by the standard stove-top method

Presoak the beans for 4 to 8 hours in ample water to cover. Drain and rinse.

Place 2 cups of water for each cup of beans in a large pot. If you wish, add a large onion, quartered, a few cloves of garlic, and 2 large bay leaves. Bring to a boil, reduce the heat, and simmer, covered, until tender, 45 to 90 minutes, depending upon the size and age of bean. Add more boiling water as needed so that the beans are always covered with liquid.

When the beans are done, drain them. Remove and discard the onion, garlic, and bay leaves if you used them. Let cool completely before dividing into portion sizes as described on page 28.

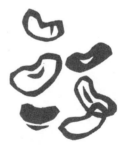

using your beans

Along with grains, beans can be the mainstay of a vegetarian diet—as they are in mine—appearing on the menu (and in this volume) in many different guises. They are more versatile than they may at first appear.

There are the obvious uses of beans—in chilies, soups, stews, and the like. Bean salads, with the addition of something crunchy such as chopped carrots, celery, or corn, make good last-minute cold entrées. Then there are the bean-based dips, spreads, and sandwich fillings that can add variety to the lunch pail.

Perhaps less obvious is the use of pureed beans to add a creamy texture to a low-fat vegetable side dish, such as Bean-Creamed Spinach (page 117), or to a cold soup like White Bean Gazpacho (page 68). For a nice change of pace, try simmering some beans in your favorite pasta sauce before ladling it over spaghetti. (See Index for more bean dishes.)

instant beans

Fantastic Foods' Instant Black and Refried Bean flakes are everything a convenience product should be: tasty, versatile, and a snap to prepare. (I'm hoping the company will soon offer an organic option.)

By following the package instructions and adding little more than boiling water, you can create a very pleasant side-dish bean puree or a filling for enchiladas. But the results are even more exciting when these precooked ground beans are used as the base for thick and satisfying soups, such as Caribbean Black Bean Soup (page 66) and Tex-Mex Pinto Soup (page 67).

Fantastic Foods' wide range of boxed products is available just about everywhere, but I find many of the company's products too salty or assertively spiced. However, the instant beans are really excellent—especially when combined with other ingredients.

going with the grains

Once you get accustomed to having whole grains in your diet, you'll miss them after a few days of pasta and white rice. Whole grains have a delightful chewiness and provide a deep sense of satisfaction. The downside is that most whole grains take a relatively long time to cook. But there's a surprising cure for that: freezing.

Cooked whole grains freeze remarkably well. This fact surprised me, too. To be honest, I had never thought of freezing grains before working on this book, assuming that they would lose taste and texture. But after a number of my recipe testers told me that they regularly added frozen cooked grains to soups and stews, I decided to give it a try.

The results were excellent, and now I always cook whole grains in large quantities, freezing what I won't use within a few days. Freeze whatever quantity of grains you have in one large Ziploc freezer bag. Although the grains freeze into a fairly solid block, banging the bag gently against the kitchen counter loosens them up and allows you to remove the amount you need. I like to keep a variety of cooked grains in the freezer, including wheat berries, kamut, barley, and brown rice. Quinoa, kasha, and oat groats don't hold up as well.

Frozen grains may be added directly to soups and stews; then simmer them until defrosted and plump, about 5 minutes. To defrost the grains separately, the microwave oven is the best bet. It does an amazing job of restoring them to their freshly cooked texture. Set them in a bowl, place a sheet of waxed paper on top of the bowl, and microwave on High for 1 to 2 minutes. You can also defrost and heat the grains right in the Ziploc freezer bag (NOT lighter-weight plastic, please!)—just make sure to open it first.

If you don't own a microwave, defrost and rehydrate the grains by placing them in a steamer basket over boiling water, covered, for 5 to 10 minutes.

whole grains under pressure

Use approximately 3 cups of water for each cup of grains. For larger quantities, increase the water by three cups for each additional cup of dry grain. *Do not fill the cooker more than halfway.*

Add 2 teaspoons of oil for every cup of dry grains.

Lock the lid in place. Bring to high pressure over high heat. Lower the heat just enough to maintain high pressure and cook for 15 minutes (brown rice, pearl barley, whole oats) or 18 minutes (kamut, Job's tears, spelt, triticale, pot barley, and rye and wheat berries).

If time permits, allow the pressure to come down naturally. Otherwise, quick-release the pressure by placing the cooker under cold running water. (Using this quick-release method avoids sputtering at the vent.) When the pressure is down, remove the lid, tilting it away from you to allow any excess steam to escape.

If the grains are not sufficiently tender—remember that whole grains are always a bit chewy—replace (but do not lock) the lid and simmer until they are done.

When, the grains are done, drain thoroughly, reserving the cooking liquid for stock if you wish. Fluff up the grains before serving. Cool leftover grains to room temperature and freeze for up to 2 months.

note: Always clean the lid, vents, and pressure regulator thoroughly after cooking grains.

presoaking grains

If you don't own a pressure cooker, a good way to cut grain cooking time by about one third is to soak the grains overnight (or all day, while you're at work) in ample water to cover by at least two inches. There's no need to drain them and add fresh water. Simply bring them to the boil in the soaking water, reduce the heat, and simmer, covered, until tender.

Cooking whole grains in a pressure cooker is a great way to get the job done quickly. Since quantity doesn't affect cooking time, make enough to store in the freezer. Grains with the same cooking times can be cooked together.

Pressure-cook whole grains in an abundance of water and then drain off the excess liquid (which you can reserve for stock). Since salt can retard the cooking time of some whole grains, I ususally add it after they are cooked tender.

To subdue the foaming action characteristic of grain cooking, always add two teaspoons of oil for every cup of dry grain. The oil prevents the grains (or loose hulls) from being catapulted into the vent, where they might interfere with the release of excess pressure. (It's best to use one of the newly designed imported cookers when cooking grains.)

Delicate and quick-cooking grains like quinoa and white rice are easily cooked by traditional stove-top methods; see the individual recipes on pages 45 and 41. One cup of dry grain yields two to two and a half cups cooked, except for barley, which yields about three and a half cups.

standard stove-top instructions for cooking whole grains

Bring a large pot of water to a boil. Add the grains and cook, covered, at a gentle boil until tender, about 30 to 45 minutes, depending on the grain. Add boiling water, if needed, to keep the grains cooking in ample liquid.

When the grains are tender, drain thoroughly, reserving the cooking liquid for stock if you wish. Fluff up the grains before serving. Cool the remainder to room temperature and freeze for up to 2 months.

quick-cooking grains

There is a handful of appealing "instant" and quick-cooking grains that invite delicious, spontaneous creations in the short-cut kitchen. These include instant polenta; whole wheat couscous; extra-long-grain, jasmine, and basmati white rice; and quinoa. I've included basic recipes here. You'll find other recipes using these grains in both the Salads and the Pasta and Grain chapters.

instant polenta

When asked to name my favorite quick-cooking grain, I'd answer "instant polenta" without hesitation. Also labeled "quick-cooking polenta" or "precooked maize meal," this wonderful product impressed me immediately with its subtle, delicious taste and smooth, soothing texture. To my mind, polenta is comfort food at its very best.

Since it cooks in under five minutes, polenta provides a terrific last-minute alternative to rice or pasta. For a quick dinner, I often serve it with a topping of chili or a cascade of chunky tomato sauce. If I'm getting really fancy, I cook polenta with frozen artichoke hearts (see page 112) or top it with a roasted portobello (see page 115).

All of the brands I've tried are imported from Italy (Valsugana and Tipiak are two I like), and use a proportion of one part polenta to four parts water. If using a brand that suggests other proportions, follow the package instructions.

basic polenta

2 cups water

Scant ½ teaspoon salt

½ teaspoon dried rosemary, oregano, or Italian herb blend (page 16 or store-bought; optional)

½ cup instant or "quick-cooking" polenta (measured into a 1-cup glass measuring cup with a pouring spout)

2 teaspoons roasted garlic or plain olive oil

prep: 2 to 3 minutes

cooking: about 3 minutes

In a medium saucepan, bring the water, rosemary (if using), and salt to a boil over high heat. Holding the measuring cup about 6 inches above the pan, gradually sprinkle in the polenta while you stir constantly and vigorously with a fork.

Reduce the heat to medium and cook, uncovered, stirring almost constantly, until the polenta thickens and loses its grittiness, 2 to 3 minutes. (When close to done, the polenta will probably begin to sputter; lower the heat and stand back.) Stir in the roasted garlic olive oil. Serve the polenta in warmed bowls.

makes 2 servings

Here's the "couldn't-be-simpler" recipe for instant polenta. You can vary it by using your favorite herbs or infused oils. Although the herbs are optional, a bit of oil is necessary to round out the polenta's flavor and texture. Cooks who use dairy products may wish to substitute two to three tablespoons of grated Parmesan cheese for the oil.

While the package instructions may tell you to cook the polenta for five minutes, I find that small amounts (half a cup of dry cornmeal or less) are done in about half the time. To avoid lumping, be sure to stir the mixture constantly while sprinkling in the polenta. In addition, hold the cornmeal well above the pot, so your arm is out of steam's reach.

Polenta squares are made by spreading hot cooked polenta into an oiled dish and letting it cool. In about fifteen minutes, the polenta firms up and you can cut it into shapes. The shaped polenta can be served at room temperature or sautéed in a little olive oil, but I prefer to grill it under the broiler. The results are crispy squares with a golden-brown crust and a creamy interior. They make attractive bases for chili, ragouts, spaghetti sauce, or greens.

It's convenient to make a double batch of Basic Polenta and turn half into shapes to refrigerate for serving later in the week.

broiled polenta squares

Vegetable oil cooking spray

1 recipe **Basic Polenta** (page 37), cooked until firm but still pourable

2 tablespoons grated **Parmesan cheese** (optional)

prep: 5 minutes

broiling: about 5 minutes

Mist an 8-inch square baking dish (or a 9-inch pie plate) with cooking spray. Pour the hot polenta into the dish. Smooth the top with a rubber spatula. Set aside, uncovered, until firm, about 15 minutes. (At this point, you may cover and refrigerate until needed, up to 5 days.)

To serve, position the broiler rack 6 inches below the element and turn on the broiler. Cut the polenta into 4 squares; if you want smaller pieces, cut each square into 2 triangles. (If using a pie plate, cut into 6 wedges.) Transfer to a lightly greased cookie sheet or the foil-covered broiler pan. Sprinkle with the Parmesan cheese (if using). Broil the polenta, without turning, until dotted with color, about 5 minutes.

makes 2 to 3 servings

whole wheat couscous

This agreeable staple of the Moroccan kitchen is now a mainstay on this side of the Atlantic, thanks to the availability of "instant" precooked varieties. (Instant couscous is popular now in Morocco too!) When whole wheat couscous showed up a few years ago, I started using this versatile grain even more often.

Whole wheat couscous is just the kind of reliable friend a hurry-up cook really appreciates: It is chameleonlike, providing a flexible background for a wide variety of flavors and ingredients. Knowing that there's some tucked away in the pantry is assurance that a delicious entrée is only minutes away.

Another great thing about couscous is that it practically cooks itself. Just pour on the boiling water, cover, and let it steep unattended while you prepare the ingredients for the rest of the dish.

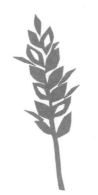

When rehydrated, couscous becomes light and fluffy, expanding to about three times its original amount.

To make fluffy couscous, ignore the often-misleading package directions and simply use roughly equal portions of water and grain. (And besides, it's much more economical to buy whole-grain couscous in bulk than in small boxes.)

Always set the couscous in a bowl or covered container and then pour the boiling water on top. Do not be tempted to bring the water to the boil in a pot and then stir in the couscous—unless you want to end up with mush. (Guess who tried doing it this way?)

When you're serving the couscous as a side-dish grain, a tablespoon of infused oil boosts the taste and improves the texture considerably.

basic whole wheat couscous

I cup whole wheat couscous

¼ teaspoon salt, or to taste

I to 1¼ cups boiling water

I tablespoon plain, roasted garlic, or basil olive oil (optional)

prep: under 5 minutes
steeping: 8 to 10 minutes

Stir the couscous and salt together in a large bowl or storage container and pour 1 cup boiling water on top. Immediately cover tightly with plastic wrap or a lid and let sit until all of the liquid is absorbed, 8 to 10 minutes. Taste, and if the couscous is not tender, stir in ¼ cup more boiling water, cover, and steep an additional 5 minutes. Fluff up with a fork. Stir in the oil if you wish.

makes about 3 cups

tasty couscous: Dress up couscous by stirring in ⅓ cup thinly sliced scallions, ¼ cup finely chopped toasted pecans or walnuts, or about 3 tablespoons minced fresh herbs.

nice white rice

White rice is one of the most easygoing foods. You could say that it has no ego: With such mild flavor and compliant texture, white rice provides an ideal backdrop, allowing the full flavor of curries and stews, for example, to stand alone in the spotlight.

My diet is quite high in fiber, so I don't hesitate to eat white rice as an occasional alternative to whole grains. I prefer fragrant basmati rice when I'm serving Indian food, or aromatic jasmine with Thai; otherwise, I use extra-long-grain Carolina.

basic white rice

2 cups water

1/2 teaspoon salt

1 cup extra-long-grain white rice

prep: 2 to 3 minutes

cooking: 18 to 20 minutes

In a medium heavy saucepan, bring the water and salt to a boil. Stir in the rice and return to a boil. Reduce the heat and simmer, covered, until all the liquid has been absorbed, 18 to 20 minutes. Fluff up before serving.

makes 3 cups

coconut rice: Add 1/3 cup unsweetened dried grated coconut along with the rice and use an extra 1/4 cup of water.

basic basmati rice

1 cup basmati rice

2 quarts water

1 teaspoon salt (optional)

prep: under 5 minutes

cooking: 10 to 12 minutes

Put the basmati in a large strainer set over a large bowl. Run water through the strainer to fill the bowl. Swish the rice a few times vigorously with your fingers and set aside to soak briefly.

Fill a large pot with the water and salt (if using) and bring to a rapid boil over high heat. When the water is boiling, lift the strainer of rice from the bowl and run cold water through it for about 10 seconds.

Stir the rice into the boiling water and cook until the rice is tender, 10 to 12 minutes. Stir occasionally, making sure that no rice is sticking to the bottom of the pot. Drain thoroughly.

Serve immediately or—for drier, fluffier rice—return the rice to the pot, cover, and let sit off the heat for 5 minutes. Fluff up before serving.

makes 3 cups

quick brown rice

Brown rice is nutritious and tasty, but it takes a solid forty-five minutes to cook (unless you use a pressure cooker). Quick Brown Rice™ from Arrowhead Mills offers a speedy twelve-minute alternative. Although the taste and texture aren't quite the same as home-cooked brown rice, it's pleasant enough and handy for last-minute meals.

basic quick brown rice

I cup Arrowhead Mills Quick Brown Rice™

I ½ cups water

¼ teaspoon salt (optional)

prep: none
cooking: 12 minutes, plus
2 minutes standing

Combine the rice, water, and salt (if using) in a medium saucepan. Bring to a boil. Reduce the heat to medium and boil, uncovered, for 10 minutes. Remove from the heat and let stand, uncovered, for 2 minutes. Fluff up and serve.

makes 2 cups

These instructions are for the Arrowhead Mills brand, which is better tasting and more economical than any other brand I've tried. According to the chart on the package, its nutritional profile is roughly equivalent to that of regular brown rice.

Quick Brown Rice™ cooks up fluffy and a bit dry, so this product works best when served with a soupy topping like curry or chili, or a stew that has lots of sauce.

quinoa

I'm crazy about this quick-cooking grain. Quinoa is actually a seed indigenous to the Andes mountains; most is still imported, but some quinoa is now grown in the Colorado Rockies. It's easy to digest and marries well with a wide variety of seasonings.

Quinoa must be thoroughly washed to remove a natural coating called saponin. Any saponin residue will give the grain a slightly bitter, grassy flavor. While many quinoa distributors wash it well, others don't—so err on the side of caution.

To rinse quinoa, set it in a large bowl and pour warm water on top. Swish vigorously. Pour into a fine-meshed strainer. Repeat the process until the water in the bowl remains fairly clear. If the quinoa was rinsed thoroughly before packaging, one round will be sufficient.

basic quinoa

1²/₃ cups water

2 teaspoons instant stock powder (optional)

¹/₂ teaspoon salt, or to taste

1 cup quinoa, thoroughly rinsed and drained (see page 44)

1 clove garlic, minced (optional)

prep: under 5 minutes

cooking: 12 to 15 minutes

In a medium heavy saucepan, bring the water, stock powder (if using), and salt to a boil over high heat. Stir in the quinoa and garlic (if using).

Cover, reduce the heat to low, and simmer until the water is absorbed and the quinoa is just tender but still crunchy, with most of the little white tails visible, about 12 minutes. If all of the liquid has been absorbed but the quinoa is not done, stir in 2 to 3 tablespoons additional boiling water, replace the cover, and simmer until the quinoa is tender, 2 to 5 minutes longer. (Alternatively, if the quinoa becomes tender before all of the liquid has been absorbed, drain the quinoa thoroughly and return to the pot to rewarm.) Fluff up before serving.

makes about 2¹/₂ cups

basic boiled quinoa: Try this foolproof technique if the above instructions are too fussy for you. Bring 2 quarts of water to a rapid boil. Add 1 teaspoon salt if you wish. Add 1 cup rinsed quinoa and cook until tender but still crunchy, about 12 minutes. Drain thoroughly.

Package instructions usually advise cooking quinoa in far too much water, resulting in a soupy porridge. Fluffy, crunchy quinoa is easy to make if you limit the amount of water and cook the grain in a heavy-bottomed pot. However, the exact cooking time and the amount of liquid required will vary slightly from batch to batch.

Adding a bit of stock powder and/or a minced clove of garlic rounds out the flavor nicely.

dips, spreads, sandwich fillings, and a quick hors d'oeuvre

This chapter brings together my tried-and-true repertoire of snack and lunch foods, from simple to sophisticated.

One of my favorite ways to create a quick and pleasing sandwich filling is to blend cooked beans with condiments or seasonings. These bean mixtures are very versatile: Thin them slightly with lemon juice or vinegar and you have a dip for chips; add some vegetable stock and leftovers become soup.

Tortilla roll-ups make a nice alternative to the standard sandwich. When company's coming, I slice these roll-ups into "sushi" for a very attractive snack or hors d'oeuvre.

Here are a few more sandwich suggestions, which make use of recipes in other chapters:

Roasted Portobello Mushrooms (page 115) on sliced foccaccia

Zesty Tofu Topping (page 122) with thinly sliced green apple or carrot on a sourdough baguette

Stir-fried vegetables (pages 97–100) stuffed into pita pockets with fresh, crispy bean sprouts

Everyone loves guacamole, but many lament its high fat content. I've come up with a good solution. My version tastes just as rich, but since pureed white beans replace some of the avocado, it weighs in much lighter.

Instead of time-consuming chopping, just blend in your favorite salsa. Depending upon the salsa you choose, the guacamole can be mellow and mild or fiery-hot.

Select a smaller, blackish bumpy-skinned Hass variety, one that is good and ripe. If time permits, allow the guacamole's flavor to develop at room temperature for fifteen minutes before serving. Have at least two limes on hand when preparing the recipe: Sometimes they are stingy with their juice!

Serve the guacamole as a dip with corn chips or raw vegetables.

dips, spreads, and fillings

quick bean guacamole

1¾ cups cooked navy beans or 1 (15-ounce) can
  navy beans, drained (rinsed if nonorganic)
1 ripe Hass avocado, halved, pitted, and the flesh
  scooped out in chunks
Approximately ¾ cup store-bought tomato salsa, preferably chunky-style
1 to 3 tablespoons freshly squeezed lime juice
Hot red pepper sauce, such as Tabasco, to taste
Salt to taste
Chopped fresh cilantro for garnish

prep: about 10 minutes
standing time (optional):
15 minutes

Place the beans, avocado chunks, ¾ cup salsa, and 1 tablespoon lime juice in the bowl of a food processor. Pulse just enough to create a coarse puree. (Or mash in a bowl with a large fork.) Add enough additional salsa and/or lime juice, hot pepper sauce, and salt to create a good balance of flavors. Transfer to a small serving bowl and garnish with cilantro.

makes 2½ cups

guacamole burritos: Roll up the guacamole in warmed flour or corn tortillas, adding a smattering of chopped tomato and minced scallion or red onion.

italian chickpea spread

1¾ cups cooked chickpeas or 1 (15-ounce) can chickpeas,
    drained (rinsed if nonorganic; reserve liquid if organic)

2 to 4 tablespoons chickpea cooking liquid (if you have it), drained
    liquid from organic canned beans, or water

1 tablespoon roasted garlic olive oil or 1 tablespoon plain olive oil
    plus 1 small clove garlic, minced

1 teaspoon Italian Herb Blend (page 16 or store-bought)

½ teaspoon salt, or to taste

1 to 3 teaspoons balsamic vinegar or freshly squeezed lemon juice
    (optional)

prep: 5 minutes

Combine the chickpeas, 2 tablespoons reserved liquid, the oil, garlic (if using), herb blend, and salt in a food processor and process until smooth, scraping down the sides of the bowl as needed. Add a bit more liquid if necessary to create a thick but spreadable consistency (or make it slightly thinner for a dip). Taste and add a little balsamic vinegar or lemon juice if you want to intensify the flavors.

makes about 1½ cups (enough for 3 hearty sandwiches)

chickpea salad dressing: Thin the spread with tomato juice (or tomato paste and water) and balsamic vinegar to taste. Add salt and freshly ground black pepper to taste.

This herby, garlicky spread has become an instant favorite. A snap to prepare, it's likely to become a staple for your lunch box. Try it on multigrain bread or stuff it into pita pockets with chopped salad greens or thinly sliced cucumbers and tomatoes. It's also good on crackers with a garnish of minced olives—or use it as a dip for raw vegetables.

Leftovers make a tasty salad dressing.

Here's a tasty way to add excitement to your lunch bag. Stuff this flavor-packed mixture into pita with thinly sliced tomato and some lettuce or sprouts, and—if you're willing to offer tastes—be prepared for lunch-mates to ask for the recipe. Try to make this the night before, as it is even tastier after a sojourn in the refrigerator. It is also delicious in Tortilla "Sushi" (page 53) or as a cracker spread or vegetable dip.

jerusalem chickpea sandwich filling

1 small rib celery, quartered, or 1 broccoli stalk, trimmed, peeled, and quartered

1¾ cups cooked chickpeas or 1 (15-ounce) can chickpeas, drained (rinsed if nonorganic)

5 to 6 tablespoons Lemon-Tahini Sauce (page 23)

2 to 3 tablespoons freshly squeezed lemon juice

½ teaspoon salt, or to taste

prep: 5 minutes (assuming already-prepared sauce)

Pulse the celery in a food processor until coarsely chopped. Add the chickpeas, 5 tablespoons sauce, 2 tablespoons lemon juice, and salt. Pulse to create a coarse puree. Taste and add more sauce, lemon juice, and/or salt as needed.

makes about 2 cups (enough for 4 sandwiches)

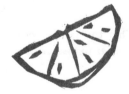

pinto salsa dip

1¾ cups cooked pinto beans or 1 (15-ounce) can
   pinto beans, drained (rinsed if nonorganic)

¾ cup store-bought fat-free salsa (mild or hot, to taste)

1 to 2 tablespoons roasted garlic olive oil or
   2 tablespoons plain olive oil plus 1 small clove garlic, minced

15 to 20 leafy sprigs cilantro

1 teaspoon salt, or to taste

Hot red pepper sauce, such as Tabasco (optional)

prep: about 5 minutes

In a food processor, pulse all of the ingredients together to create a fairly smooth puree. Taste and adjust the seasoning. Transfer to a serving bowl.

makes 1½ cups

Combining beans with salsa creates a creamy, flavor-packed dip—but since the flavor relies almost entirely on the salsa, be sure to use one you know and love. The pintos mellow the salsa's heat, so opt for a spicier variety than you'd normally choose, or "zip it up" with a little Tabasco after blending.

This recipe was developed using a fat-free salsa. If your salsa contains oil and sufficient garlic, taste the dip before adding the garlic-infused olive oil.

Serve the dip in a bowl accompanied by corn chips. Stuff leftovers into pita pockets with cubed avocado.

For another interesting approach to the bean-salsa theme, take a look at the Black Bean–Tomato Salsa Salad on page 76.

red pepper hummus

1¾ cups cooked chickpeas or 1 (15-ounce) can   **prep:** under 10 minutes
   chickpeas, drained (rinsed if nonorganic; reserve
   liquid if organic)

½ cup diced roasted red pepper (page 9 or store-bought)

3 tablespoons sesame tahini

2 tablespoons freshly squeezed lemon juice, or more to taste

1 tablespoon olive oil

1 large clove garlic, halved

2 teaspoons ground coriander

1 teaspoon cumin seeds

1 teaspoon *harissa* or ⅛ teaspoon cayenne, or more to taste

1 teaspoon salt, or more to taste

Oil-cured black olives for garnish (optional)

Place all of the ingredients (except the olives) in the bowl of a food processor and process until smooth. If the mixture seems too thick, blend in 1 to 3 tablespoons of the reserved chickpea liquid or water to create the desired consistency. (It should be fairly thick for a sandwich filling, thinner for a dip.) Taste and add more lemon juice, *harissa*, and/or salt if needed. Transfer to a bowl and garnish with olives if you like.

makes about 1¾ cups

parsley hummus: Substitute the leaves from a small bunch of parsley for the roasted pepper.

low-fat hummus: Omit the tahini and olive oil and substitute 1 to 2 teaspoons toasted sesame oil.

a quick hors d'oeuvre

tortilla "sushi"

1 recipe Spinach Pesto (page 107),
   Red Pepper Hummus (page 52),
   Italian Chickpea Spread (page 49), or
   Jerusalem Chickpea Sandwich Filling (page 50)

5 whole wheat tortillas (about 7 inches in diameter)

½ cup diced roasted red peppers (page 9 or store-bought) or chopped fresh basil

prep: under 10 minutes (assuming already-prepared filling)

Place about ⅓ cup of the filling on each tortilla and pat it into an even layer, leaving a ½-inch arch across the top free of filling. Scatter about 2 tablespoons roasted pepper or basil leaves over the filling. Roll up tightly and press the top edge gently into place to seal it.

If heating, place the rolls on a nonstick cookie sheet and bake at 350 degrees until warm throughout, about 10 minutes.

To slice, use a gentle sawing action with a serrated knife: Trim off the ends and cut into slices about 1 inch thick. For a more unusual look, alternate making slices straight down and slices on the diagonal to create pieces about 1½ inches on the long side and ½ inch on the short. Set flat sides down to serve.

makes about 30 pieces

mountain sushi: Use the relatively new product called Mountain Bread instead of tortillas. These breads are the same size and shape as tortillas but come in a tasty multigrain version.

I'm normally not one to fuss with finger food hors d'oeuvres, but making attractive tortilla "sushi" is easy and fun—and they look very pretty. To make them, you simply spread one of the fillings listed below over a large whole wheat tortilla, dot it with diced roasted red pepper or fresh basil leaves to add some color, roll it up, and slice.

If you're serving the sushi as an appetizer or cocktail snack, allow three to four slices per person. Those made with the chickpea-based filling are good at room temperature, but those with the spinach pesto are better warm. For an attractive presentation, set the sushi on a bed of radicchio or watercress.

soups for supper

(and lunch too)

Ah, soup. I know it's fall when I reach for the soup pot. Somehow, as the air gets cooler and the days shorter, I always take comfort in warming myself up with a steaming bowlful.

I like my soups thick and hearty—the kind I can make an entire meal of—with perhaps a slice of crusty bread and a salad or slaw. Besides, when I'm in short-cut mode, I'm not likely to prepare more than one course. For that reason, for a few of the soups that are light enough to serve as appetizers, I've also offered instructions for turning them into entrées.

The quickest way to make a great-tasting soup is to use the pressure cooker, where flavors mingle in record time. I've given optional pressure-cooker instructions where appropriate for those of you who own one. But primarily these recipes show you other ways to prepare soups that offer very good taste with only a small investment of preparation and cooking time.

quick-cooking mushroom-barley soup

1 tablespoon olive or canola oil

1 1/2 cups coarsely chopped onions or
    thinly sliced leeks

1 1/2 teaspoons minced garlic

6 cups boiling water

1/4 cup tomato paste

3 tablespoons instant vegetable stock powder

Generous 1/2 cup quick-cooking barley

1/2 ounce sliced dried mushrooms (about 1/2 cup), quickly rinsed or
    reconstituted if sandy (see page 9)

3 large carrots, trimmed and cut into 1/4-inch slices

2 large ribs celery, trimmed and cut into 1/4-inch slices

2 to 3 teaspoons dried dill

1/2 teaspoon dried thyme

1/2 teaspoon salt, or to taste

2 to 4 tablespoons dry sherry or 1 to 2 teaspoons balsamic vinegar
    (optional)

Freshly ground black pepper to taste

prep: about 15 minutes

cooking: 15 to 25 minutes

In a large soup pot, heat the oil over medium heat. Sauté the onions and garlic for 1 minute, stirring frequently. Add the boiling water, tomato paste, stock powder, barley, mushrooms, carrots, celery, 2 teaspoons dill, the

Most New Yorkers have heard of Ratners, the bastion of Russian Jewish cooking on the Lower East Side. There they serve a grandma-style mushroom-barley soup that brings tears of nostalgia to my eyes. With the help of quick-cooking barley and dried mushrooms, I've created a beat-the-clock version of this timeless classic.

The soup is tasty after about fifteen minutes of cooking, but if you have time to simmer it for ten minutes longer, you'll get that wonderful creamy thickness that is the essence of any great mushroom-barley soup. To complete the Ratners experience, serve the soup with fresh onion rolls.

thyme, and salt. Stir well and bring to a boil. Cover, lower the heat, and simmer for 5 minutes. Taste and add up to 1 teaspoon more dill if you like. Cover and simmer until the vegetables and barley are tender, about 5 more minutes. If you wish, enhance the flavor with either sherry or balsamic vinegar, and add black pepper to taste.

makes 5 to 6 servings

short-cut soup tips

- **For optimum taste, make sure to use high-quality instant vegetable stock powder (see page 14) and organic canned beans.**
- **To cut down on cooking time, bring the water to a boil in a kettle while you are chopping the vegetables and doing any initial sautéing. Then add the boiling water to the soup pot.**
- **Finely chopped vegetables cook much more quickly than larger pieces.**
- **Chop vegetables of similar density together in the food processor.**
- **Buy peeled and trimmed baby carrots.**
- **To avoid slowing down the cooking process, defrost frozen vegetables before adding them to the soup.**
- **Use quick-cooking creamy thickeners such as oatmeal, potato flakes, quick-cooking barley, and instant bean flakes.**

butternut squash soup with herbes de provence

2 pounds butternut squash, peeled, seeded,
    and cut into 1½-inch chunks

2 large ribs celery, cut into 2-inch pieces

1 tablespoon olive oil

1½ cups thinly sliced leeks (white and light green parts only) or
    coarsely chopped onions

3 cups water

1½ tablespoons instant vegetable stock powder

⅓ cup old-fashioned rolled oats

2 teaspoons Herbes de Provence (page 17 or store-bought)

½ teaspoon salt, or more to taste

2 to 3 teaspoons sherry vinegar or balsamic vinegar

¼ cup snipped fresh chives or thinly sliced scallion greens, for garnish

prep: about 15 minutes
cooking: 15 minutes

Using the food processor, finely chop the squash in several batches. (You should have about 5 cups.) Transfer to a large bowl. Finely chop the celery. Set aside with the squash.

In a large soup pot, heat the oil and sauté the leeks for 1 minute. Add the water and stock powder and bring to a boil over high heat. Stir in the squash, celery, oats, herbes de Provence, and salt and return to a boil. Reduce the heat to medium, cover, and cook at a gentle boil until the squash is very soft, about 15 minutes.

Puree the soup with an immersion blender (or cool slightly, then transfer in small batches to a food processor or blender and blend until smooth).

This burnished-orange soup has a silken texture and a beautiful sheen, thanks to the addition of oatmeal—a terrific short-cut technique for creating quick body and creaminess. Chopping the squash and celery very finely in the food processor dramatically reduces cooking time without forsaking full-bodied taste. Be sure to include the chive (or scallion) garnish, which adds dramatic visual and flavor contrast. If you like, stir in a tablespoon of basil or rosemary olive oil at the end for an additional flavor dimension.

Accompany the soup with focaccia and a salad or steamed green vegetable to make a wholesome and colorful meal.

Stir in enough vinegar to heighten the flavors. Add a bit more salt if needed, and reheat if necessary. Garnish with the chives.

makes 4 servings

cooking under pressure: After the initial sauté, cook all the ingredients in a pressure cooker for 4 minutes under high pressure. Use a quick-release method or allow the pressure to come down naturally. Proceed as directed in the recipe.

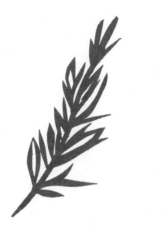

The combination of curry and coconut is a tradition in Indian cooking for good reason: It's terrific. (But do be sure that your curry powder is fresh, or make your own as described on page 17.) I've had great results making this soup with Merwanjee Poonjiajee & Sons Madras curry powder. The sweetness—and bright orange color—of the carrots and the fragrance of the coconut milk are also memorable components of this smooth, elegant soup.

To reduce prep time, use baby carrots (which, by the way, are usually peeled mature carrots trimmed and shaped to look like baby ones).

curried carrot soup

2½ cups water

1 (14-ounce) can coconut milk (not "lite")

1 heaping tablespoon instant vegetable stock powder

1 tablespoon plus 1 teaspoon mild curry blend (page 17 or store-bought)

½ teaspoon salt, or more to taste

1 pound carrots, peeled or scrubbed, trimmed and cut into large chunks, or baby carrots

1 large sweet onion (about 8 ounces), quartered

1 large russet potato (about 8 ounces), peeled and cut into 8 chunks

Finely chopped fresh cilantro for garnish (optional)

prep: about 10 minutes (if using baby carrots)

cooking: 20 minutes

In a large soup pot, bring the water, coconut milk, stock powder, curry, and salt to a boil over high heat.

Meanwhile, in several batches, pulse the carrots, onion, and potato in a food processor until very finely chopped. As you finish chopping each batch, add it to the soup. Return the soup to a boil, cover, and simmer, stirring occasionally, until the carrots are very soft, about 20 minutes.

Puree the soup with an immersion blender (or cool slightly and puree in small batches in a blender or food processor). Add more salt if needed and reheat if necessary. Garnish each serving with cilantro if you wish.

makes 4 servings

cooking under pressure: Leave the carrots in large chunks but coarsely chop the onion and potato. Cook the soup in a pressure cooker for 5 minutes under high pressure. Use a quick-release method or allow the pressure to come down naturally. Proceed as directed in the recipe.

curried carrot and pea soup with basmati rice: Turn leftovers into a main dish by reheating with some frozen peas. Ladle the soup over boiled basmati rice and garnish with a sprinkling of finely chopped cilantro.

green leek and potato soup

2 tablespoons roasted garlic olive oil or
    1 tablespoon each roasted garlic and basil
    or rosemary olive oil

prep: under 10 minutes
cooking: under 15 minutes

3 cups thinly sliced leeks (white and light green parts), separated into
    rings, thoroughly rinsed, and drained

4 cups boiling water

1½ tablespoons instant vegetable stock powder

¾ teaspoon salt, or to taste

1 (10-ounce) package frozen chopped spinach

1 cup unseasoned instant mashed potato flakes (Barbara's are good)

Freshly ground black pepper to taste

3 tablespoons minced fresh parsley, for garnish (optional)

In a soup pot, heat 1 tablespoon roasted garlic oil and sauté the leeks, stirring frequently, until they begin to brown, about 3 minutes. Add the boiling water, stock powder, and salt and bring to a boil. Add the spinach, cover, and cook, occasionally breaking up the block of spinach with a fork, until the spinach is cooked but still bright green, 5 to 8 minutes.

Turn the heat down to a simmer and sprinkle in the potato flakes while you stir. The soup will thicken almost immediately. Add black pepper to taste and the additional tablespoon of infused olive oil. Sprinkle each serving with the parsley if you wish.

makes 2 hearty servings

green leek, potato, and corn soup: Add 1 cup of defrosted corn kernels along with the potato flakes.

leek and potato soup with fresh chard: Omit the spinach and add ½ pound Swiss chard, trimmed and finely chopped. Cook until the chard is tender, 3 to 5 minutes, before adding the potato flakes.

There is nothing like a good leek and potato soup, with its mellow texture and harmonious flavors. It feels like magic to be able to produce such a satisfying rendition of this timeless recipe in a matter of minutes.

My secret weapon is instant potato flakes. Just stir them in and watch the soup develop a creamy thickness and a distinctive potato flavor in about thirty seconds. While I wouldn't rave about instant mashed potatoes, the flakes are surprisingly delicious in this thick soup.

What about the green in the recipe's title? I've taken the liberty of tampering with the classic components by adding spinach, which gives the soup a whole new dimension—plus cheerful flecks of verdant color.

miso vegetable hot pot

6 cups water

3 tablespoons instant vegetable stock powder

½ to ¾ pound firm tofu, drained and diced

½ to ¾ pound bok choy, trimmed and thinly sliced

1 (8-ounce) can sliced baby corn, drained and rinsed

Approximately 3 tablespoons dark miso, such as barley or hatcho

½ cup thinly sliced scallion greens

Toasted sesame oil to taste (optional)

prep: about 10 minutes
cooking: under 5 minutes

In a large soup pot, bring the water and stock powder to a boil over high heat. Ladle about ½ cup of the hot liquid into a 2-cup glass measuring cup and set aside.

Add the tofu, bok choy, and baby corn to the pot and simmer, covered, over medium-high heat for 2 minutes. Meanwhile, dissolve 3 tablespoons miso in the reserved hot liquid by stirring vigorously with a fork and mashing the miso against the side of the cup.

When the bok choy is tender but the stems still have some crunch, turn off the heat. Stir in the miso solution, the scallion greens, and sesame oil to taste (if using). If the broth isn't flavorful enough, add a tablespoon more miso (first dissolving it in ¼ cup of the cooking liquid). Reheat if necessary. Serve in large soup bowls.

makes 4 hearty servings

Here are some good ways to vary the hot pot:

- Use a different miso or combine two types of miso—light and dark.
- For a burst of flavor, add a tablespoon of grated fresh ginger to the soup—or stir in about ¼ cup of minced cilantro at the end.
- For more crunch, about a minute before the soup is done, add 3 ounces snow peas, trimmed and cut into 1-inch slices on the diagonal, and/or 1 small carrot, trimmed, halved lengthwise, and thinly sliced.
- For a briny flavor, add 1 to 2 tablespoons of instant wakame sea vegetable along with the bok choy.
- Add a cup or two of cooked grains, but stir well before serving, as they tend to sink to the bottom of the pot.

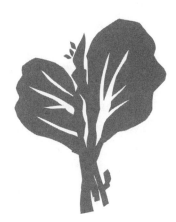

With all of these possibilities, you might find the soup getting too chock-full of ingredients. If so, just dissolve additional miso in boiling water—about a heaping teaspoon per each cup—and stir it in.

provençal red lentil soup

The aroma of the herbes de Provence in this simple but substantial soup will transport you to a sunny garden in the South of France. Although the soup has no oil, the smooth texture of the red lentils gives it a creamy richness. To enhance this aspect, you can puree all or part of the soup. Red lentils are a "primo" short-cut legume because they cook so quickly and require no presoaking.

Serve the soup with a sliced baguette so you and your guests can mop up every last drop.

5 cups water

1 heaping tablespoon instant vegetable stock powder

1 cup red lentils, picked over and rinsed

2 cups chopped leeks (white and light green parts only) or onions

3 large carrots, peeled or scrubbed, trimmed, halved lengthwise, and cut into ½-inch slices, or 8 baby carrots, cut into 1-inch chunks

1½ teaspoons Herbes de Provence (page 17 or store-bought)

Salt and freshly ground black pepper to taste

2 tablespoons chopped fresh parsley, for garnish (optional)

prep: 10 minutes
cooking: about 20 minutes

In a heavy soup pot, bring the water and stock powder to a boil. Add the lentils (if they've stuck together after rinsing, separate them with a fork), leeks, carrots, and herbs. Return to a boil, then reduce the heat and simmer, covered, until the lentils are very soft, about 20 minutes. Stir frequently and well, as the lentils tend to sink to the bottom.

Stir in salt and pepper to taste, garnish with parsley if you wish, and serve.

makes 4 servings

cooking under pressure: Add 1 tablespoon of olive oil along with the lentils and cook in a pressure cooker for 4 minutes under high pressure. Allow the pressure to come down naturally or use a quick-release method. Stir well and add salt and pepper to taste.

mediterranean white bean soup with escarole

1 tablespoon roasted garlic or plain olive oil

1 cup thinly sliced leeks or coarsely chopped
    onions

1¾ cups cooked navy or cannellini beans or 1 (15-ounce) can navy or
    cannellini beans, drained (rinsed if nonorganic)

1 (14.5-ounce) can crushed tomatoes

2 cups boiling water

1 tablespoon instant vegetable stock powder

1 teaspoon Italian Herb Blend (page 16 or store-bought)

½ teaspoon salt, or to taste

½ pound escarole, leaves separated and thoroughly rinsed

A few tablespoons of grated Parmesan cheese or
    1 to 2 teaspoons balsamic vinegar

Freshly ground black pepper to taste

1 tablespoon basil olive oil or ¼ cup chopped fresh basil

prep: under 15 minutes
cooking: about 10 minutes

In this robust soup, the Italian seasoning blend offers an herbal backdrop to the traditional Mediterranean combination of greens and white beans. The white beans give the soup a slow-cooked, mellow texture, offset by the escarole's slightly bitter edge. I like to enhance the soup with either basil-infused olive oil or fresh basil.

In a large soup pot, heat the oil and sauté the leeks for 1 minute, stirring frequently. Add the beans, tomatoes, boiling water, stock powder, herbs, and salt and bring to a boil over high heat.

While the soup is coming to the boil, stack the escarole leaves and coarsely chop them. (Or chop them in several batches in a food processor.) You should have 7 to 8 loosely packed cups.

When the soup is boiling, stir in the escarole. Cook over medium heat, uncovered, stirring occasionally, until the escarole is tender, 8 to 10 minutes. Season to taste with the Parmesan or balsamic vinegar and pepper. Stir in the basil olive oil or fresh basil just before serving.

makes 2 to 3 servings

No one who tastes this soup will believe it when you confess (if you do confess) that it takes only ten minutes to prepare from start to finish. I think you'll be amazed by the dense flavor and silken smoothness that result from combining coconut milk and instant black beans.

For a heartier version, add about one cup each of cooked rice and corn (fresh or frozen). Either Asian Slaw or Moroccan Carrot Slaw (page 81 or 83) offers a good contrast of taste and texture.

caribbean black bean soup

2½ cups water

1 (14-ounce) can "lite" coconut milk

1 (14.5-ounce) can diced tomatoes with
   green chilies or 1 (14.5-ounce) can diced tomatoes plus 1 large
   jalapeño, seeded and thinly sliced

1 (7-ounce) package Fantastic Foods Instant Black Beans

Salt to taste

Hot red pepper sauce, such as Tabasco, to taste

¼ cup chopped fresh cilantro, for garnish

prep: 5 minutes

cooking: about 3 minutes,
plus 5 minutes standing

In a soup pot, bring the water, coconut milk, and tomatoes (with canning liquid) to a boil over high heat, stirring often. Stir in the instant black beans and season with salt and hot pepper sauce. Cover, turn off the heat, and let stand for 5 minutes. Stir well and reheat if necessary. Serve in soup bowls, garnished with the cilantro.

makes 4 servings

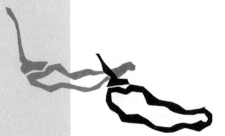

tex-mex pinto soup

1 tablespoon olive oil

1 cup coarsely chopped onions

1 tablespoon minced garlic

1 large jalapeño, seeded and diced, or ¼ teaspoon crushed red pepper
   flakes

1½ teaspoons cumin seeds

4 cups water

1 (7-ounce) package Fantastic Foods Instant Refried Beans

Salt to taste

1 cup fresh or frozen corn (no need to defrost)

¼ cup minced fresh cilantro

prep: under 10 minutes

cooking: under 10 minutes

Heat the oil in a heavy soup pot. Sauté the onions, garlic, jalapeño, and cumin for 1 minute, stirring frequently. Add the water and bring to a boil. Whisk in the bean flakes and salt to taste. Cover, reduce the heat, and simmer for 4 minutes.

Stir in the corn and cook, uncovered, until the corn is tender, 1 to 2 minutes. Stir in the cilantro just before serving.

makes 3 to 4 servings

tex-mex black bean soup: Substitute Fantastic Foods Instant Black Beans for the Refried Beans.

This is an easy soup to prepare, but that doesn't mean it's bland. Some of the robust seasoning comes right along with the instant refried beans. I've spiked it up with southwestern accents such as jalapeño, cumin, and cilantro, and added a good supply of onions and corn.

To make it even more rib-sticking, stir one and a half cups cooked quinoa into the finished soup. (Thin it with a little stock or water if it gets too thick.) If you like, sprinkle each portion with regular or soy-based shredded Cheddar or Monterey Jack. Serve the soup with heated tortillas or corn chips.

For a refreshing summer appetizer—or light main dish, if served in larger amounts—gazpacho can't be beat. In this unorthodox version, pureed white beans create a low-fat soup that nevertheless seems rich and creamy. If you plan ahead and chill the canned beans and tomatoes, you won't even have to chill the finished soup.

If you can find them, use Kirby (pickling) cucumbers. They are smaller, denser, and more flavorful than the large waxed supermarket variety, and their unwaxed skins don't require peeling. If using fresh tomatoes, you may need to thin the soup slightly with canned tomato juice or water.

white bean gazpacho

1 (15-ounce) can navy beans
(preferably organic; see Note)
1 small clove garlic
2 to 3 teaspoons sherry vinegar or red wine vinegar
1 (14.5-ounce) can diced tomatoes with green chilies or 1½ to 2 cups
seeded and finely diced plum tomatoes plus 1 jalapeño,
seeded and diced
1 cup diced cucumbers, preferably Kirby (pickling) cucumbers
Salt to taste
Hot red pepper sauce, such as Tabasco, to taste

prep: under 10 minutes
chilling time: 30 minutes (or much less if ingredients are prechilled)

In a food processor, puree the beans with their liquid (or the tomato juice; see Note), the garlic, and 2 teaspoons vinegar until very smooth. If you're using fresh tomatoes, add half of them plus the diced jalapeño at this point. Transfer to a bowl. Stir in the canned tomatoes, or the remaining fresh, the cucumbers, and a bit more vinegar if needed, to give the soup a slight acid edge. Add salt and hot pepper sauce to taste. Serve chilled.

note: If you're not using organic beans, drain and rinse them. Substitute ½ cup tomato juice for the canned bean liquid.

makes 3 to 4 servings

roasted red pepper gazpacho: Puree ⅓ cup diced roasted red pepper (page 9 or store-bought) along with the beans. Proceed as directed in the recipe.

herbed white bean gazpacho: Stir in 1 tablespoon rosemary or basil olive oil at the end, or drizzle a bit over each serving.

salads in the limelight,

salads on the side

I enjoy inventing salads just about as much as I enjoy inventing soups. Both categories invite the spontaneous tossing together of ingredients— combining what's on hand in the pantry with what's in season at the produce stand.

I often serve grain- or bean-based salads as entrées. They are pretty, filling, and easy to make ahead. In fact, they usually taste better after marinating in the dressing for a few hours.

Certainly the simplest entrée salads to create are those based on whole wheat couscous. While this "instant" grain is briefly steeping in boiling water, you have just enough time to prepare the remaining ingredients. Because couscous is so light, it usually comes to mind in warm weather, or when I'm serving the salad for lunch.

I turn to Whole-Grain Tabbouleh or Grain Salad with Lemon-Tahini Sauce when I'm looking for something heartier. The preparation of these is streamlined when you've prepared leftover grains on purpose or defrosted a portion of cooked grains previously stashed in the freezer (see page 34).

As you'll read elsewhere in this book, I'm a great fan of cabbage, and, not surprisingly, one of my favorite side salads is slaw. The three cabbage slaws in this chapter demonstrate the diversity you can achieve by changing the accompanying ingredients and coating the slaw with different dressings. Almost any hard vegetable that's good raw can be transformed into a crunchy, colorful slaw, and I've included a Moroccan carrot version just to prove my point.

grain salads

whole-grain tabbouleh

3 cups cooked whole grains (such as kamut,
　wheat berries, or brown rice)

2 cups seeded and diced plum tomatoes

2 cups peeled, seeded, and diced cucumbers, preferably Kirby pickling
　cucumbers (see Note)

1 cup finely chopped fresh parsley

½ cup finely chopped red onion

⅓ cup finely chopped fresh mint or 1 to 2 teaspoons dried mint

3 tablespoons roasted garlic oil, or 3 tablespoons plain olive oil
　plus 1 to 2 small cloves garlic, minced

3 to 5 tablespoons freshly squeezed lemon juice

1 teaspoon salt, or to taste

Freshly ground black pepper to taste

prep: 15 minutes (assuming already-cooked grains)

In a large bowl or storage container, combine the grains, tomatoes, cucumbers, parsley, onion, and mint. Drizzle the oil and 3 tablespoons lemon juice over the mixture while you stir. Add the salt, pepper, and additional lemon juice if necessary to give the salad a nice puckery edge.

note: I prefer small Kirby cucumbers since they are less watery than large cucumbers. Because they're not waxed, Kirbys don't have to be peeled—just scrubbed.

makes 4 to 6 main-course servings

Here's a twist on the traditional Middle Eastern tabbouleh, using whole grains instead of bulgur. Because of the whole grains, this salad is chewier and more filling than a typical tabbouleh.

I especially like to prepare whole-grain tabbouleh with kamut, a large golden grain with lots of character and a buttery taste. You'll also have good results with wheat berries, brown rice, barley, or a combination of whatever cooked or frozen grains (see page 34) you have on hand.

To dress it up, serve the tabbouleh on a bed of radicchio, garnished with fresh orange segments and some good Mediterranean olives. If you have any leftovers, perk them up with a bit more lemon juice just before serving.

A delicious parsley-flecked tahini dressing pairs well with grains, currants, and carrots to create a festive and unusual salad. Try it with kamut, brown rice, or barley—or a combination of whatever freshly cooked or defrosted frozen grains (see page 34) you have on hand. Avoid white rice, though, since it is too delicate to support the creamy, tangy sauce.

This salad is hearty enough to make a meal, especially if you expand it with a cup or two of finely chopped cooked kale or collard greens. (If you do, add a little more of that great sauce.) Alternatively, serve it on a bed of raw spinach, garnished with sliced tomatoes and warmed pita wedges.

grain salad with lemon-tahini sauce

3 cups cooked whole grains

1 cup finely chopped carrots

⅓ cup dried currants

½ cup thinly sliced scallion greens

5 to 6 tablespoons Lemon-Tahini Sauce (page 23)

Freshly squeezed lemon juice to taste

Salt to taste

prep: 10 minutes (assuming already-cooked grains)

In a large bowl or storage container, combine the grains, carrots, currants, and scallions. Toss in enough dressing to thoroughly coat the grains. Add enough lemon juice and salt to give the salad a vibrant taste.

makes 4 main-course servings

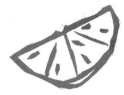

arame-flecked asian couscous

1½ cups whole wheat couscous

1 tablespoon minced fresh ginger

⅛ teaspoon cayenne

1½ to 1¾ cups boiling water

½ ounce arame sea vegetable (about 1 cup loosely packed)

1½ cups finely chopped carrots

1 cup finely chopped radishes

¾ cup thinly sliced scallion greens

2 to 3 tablespoons toasted sesame oil

3 to 4 tablespoons shoyu or tamari

Approximately 3 tablespoons brown rice or seasoned rice vinegar
   (the latter adds sweetness too)

⅓ cup toasted sunflower seeds

prep: 15 minutes

Steeping: about 10 minutes

Mix the couscous, ginger, and cayenne in a large heatproof bowl or storage container and pour 1½ cups boiling water on top. Cover tightly and let sit until all of the liquid is absorbed, about 10 minutes. If the couscous is not quite tender, stir in an additional ¼ cup boiling water, cover, and let sit for a few minutes longer. Fluff up with a fork, and let cool.

Meanwhile, place the arame in a bowl with ample cold water to cover and let stand until rehydrated, about 10 minutes. Rinse thoroughly and drain well.

Add the drained arame, carrots, radishes, and scallions to the couscous. Stir in enough sesame oil, shoyu, and vinegar to give the salad intense flavor. Stir in the sunflower seeds. Serve at room temperature. (Leftovers will probably need to be perked up with additional dressing.)

makes 4 main-course servings

When it comes to flavorings, most recipes keep couscous firmly planted in the Mediterranean. But because of its mild flavor and versatility, couscous has tempted me to embark on taste adventures farther afield.

In this visually striking salad, couscous is flecked with another easily prepared ingredient: arame, an elegant, jet-black mildly briny sea vegetable used in Japanese cooking. Arame is ready to eat after a brief soak in water. Asian seasonings integrate the couscous and arame in a memorable way.

Use a food processor to chop the carrots and radishes while the couscous is steeping. Serve the salad on a bed of watercress, garnished with some cherry tomatoes or sliced kumquats.

This salad—named for the Mexican seasonings and the combination of black beans and corn—is gorgeous to behold, with its flecks of black, yellow, red, and green. It is even more dramatic when set atop a bed of radicchio or watercress. Garnish the salad with sliced avocados and cherry tomatoes—or dice a cupful of either and toss right in.

aztec couscous

1 cup whole wheat couscous

½ teaspoon ground cumin

1 teaspoon salt, or to taste

1 to 1¼ cups boiling water

1¾ cups cooked black beans or 1 (15-ounce) can black beans, drained (rinsed if nonorganic)

1 cup fresh corn, cooked, or defrosted frozen corn

½ cup finely diced red onion

¼ cup finely minced fresh cilantro

1 jalapeño pepper, seeded and diced (optional)

2 tablespoons roasted garlic olive oil

3 to 4 tablespoons freshly squeezed lime juice

prep: under 15 minutes

steeping: about 10 minutes

Place the couscous, cumin, and salt in a large heatproof bowl or storage container and pour 1 cup boiling water on top. Cover tightly and let sit until all of the liquid is absorbed, about 10 minutes. If the couscous is not quite tender, stir in an additional ¼ cup boiling water, cover, and let sit for a few minutes longer. Fluff up with a fork.

Toss in the beans, corn, onion, cilantro, and jalapeño (if using). Mix in the olive oil and enough lime juice to give the salad a puckery edge. Serve warm or at room temperature.

makes 4 main-course servings

quinoa-corn salad with basil

5 cups water

1 teaspoon salt, or more to taste

1½ cups quinoa, thoroughly rinsed and
  drained (see page 45)

2 cups fresh corn, cooked, or defrosted frozen corn

1 cup tightly packed fresh basil leaves, finely chopped

½ cup diced roasted red peppers (page 9 or store-bought)

½ cup finely diced red onions

2 tablespoons plain or roasted garlic olive oil

3 to 5 tablespoons freshly squeezed lemon juice

prep: 5 minutes
cooking: about 12 minutes
cooling: under 15 minutes

In a medium saucepan, bring the water and salt to a rolling boil over high heat. Stir in the quinoa. Return to a boil, reduce the heat to medium, and cook at a gentle boil for 11 minutes.

Add the corn and continue to cook until the quinoa is tender but still crunchy, 1 to 3 more minutes. Drain thoroughly.

Transfer the quinoa to a serving bowl or storage container. Stir to fluff it up and to release excess heat. Set aside until cooled to room temperature.

Stir in the basil, red peppers, onions, and olive oil. Add salt, if needed, and enough lemon juice to give the salad a distinct lemony edge. (Leftovers will probably need to be perked up with additional lemon juice.)

makes 4 main-course servings

This salad is a delight to make in the summer, when fresh basil and corn are in abundance. If you're a newcomer to quinoa, this is a good recipe to try: Quinoa and corn are natural partners. You'll have time to prepare the basil, red pepper, and onion while the quinoa is cooling.

For a striking presentation, serve the salad inside hollowed-out beefsteak tomatoes.

black bean–tomato salsa salad

Is it a salad or is it a salsa? This spicy dish is too good to be pigeonholed. You can present it in a bowl as a dip for corn chips, but it certainly makes a noteworthy luncheon or light supper entrée—mounded into a radicchio cup.

There are a number of simple ways to vary this recipe: You can use basil instead of cilantro, stir in one cup defrosted frozen corn kernels or cooked rice, or add one tablespoon roasted garlic oil or one minced garlic clove.

For optimum taste, assemble the salad at least half an hour before serving.

1¾ cups cooked black beans or 1 (15-ounce) can black beans, drained (rinsed if nonorganic)

1 (14.5-ounce) can diced tomatoes with green chilies, drained, or 1½ cups finely diced plum tomatoes plus 1 jalapeño, seeded and minced

½ cup finely minced red onion or scallions

⅓ to ½ cup minced fresh cilantro (depending on how much you like it)

3 to 4 tablespoons freshly squeezed lime juice

½ teaspoon salt, or to taste

prep: 10 minutes
marinating: at least 30 minutes

In a bowl or storage container, toss together the beans, tomatoes, onion, cilantro, 3 tablespoons lime juice, and the salt. Let sit at room temperature for at least 30 minutes.

Just before serving, taste and add extra lime juice if desired.

makes 2 main-course servings or 4 to 6 servings as dip

bonus jalapeño-tomato salad dressing: If you use canned diced tomatoes with green chilies, don't discard the drained juice! Combine it with 1 tablespoon olive oil, 2 tablespoons freshly squeezed lemon juice, and 1½ teaspoons tamari for a zesty salad dressing.

pinto bean salad with lemony maple-mustard dressing

1¾ cups cooked pinto beans or 1 (15-ounce)
   can pinto beans, drained (rinsed if
   nonorganic)

1½ cups fresh corn, cooked, or defrosted frozen corn

½ cup finely diced red bell pepper or roasted red pepper
   (page 9 or store-bought)

½ cup thinly sliced scallion greens

⅓ cup Lemony Maple-Mustard Dressing (page 21)

Tamari to taste (optional)

Freshly squeezed lemon juice to taste (optional)

prep: 10 minutes
marinating: 10 to 15 minutes
(or longer if you wish)

In a large bowl or storage container, combine the beans, corn, bell pepper, and scallions. Add the dressing and toss to coat. If time permits, set aside to allow the beans to absorb the dressing, 10 to 15 minutes, or longer.

Taste before serving: If the salad seems a little bland, add a bit of tamari and/or stir in lemon juice to create a vibrant flavor.

makes 3 to 4 main-course servings

pinto salad in a "bowl": Mound the salad into and over "bowls" of halved, pitted avocados or hollowed-out beefsteak tomatoes. Place on a bed of greens that have been lightly coated with Very Versatile Vinaigrette (page 19).

This salad relies on a zippy dressing that has two noteworthy things going for it: It's fat-free, and it does an admirable job of livening up mild-mannered pintos. Indeed, the mixture tastes best if the beans have had a chance to absorb the dressing, so do try to make it at least an hour ahead.

The salad works well as part of a buffet or picnic ensemble that might include Whole-Grain Tabbouleh (page 71) and Moroccan Carrot Slaw (page 83). It's especially popular with kids.

dilled cauliflower salad

Here's an unusual salad I like to make in the microwave, which does a remarkable job of taking the raw edge off cauliflower while leaving its crunch and appealing, subtle flavor intact. (I've included standard cooking instructions for those who don't own a microwave.)

The simple dressing of dill, olive oil, and lemon juice brings out the best in this often overlooked vegetable. Indeed, this recipe is likely to make some new cauliflower converts. When they're in season, small cherry tomatoes make a nice addition to the salad.

2 tablespoons water

6 cups small cauliflower florets (1 ½ inches across the top) (about 1 pound)

1 small red onion, coarsely chopped

1 teaspoon dried dill

2 tablespoons roasted garlic olive oil or 2 tablespoons plain olive oil plus 1 to 2 small cloves garlic, minced

2 tablespoons freshly squeezed lemon juice, or more to taste

½ teaspoon salt

Freshly ground black pepper to taste

prep: under 10 minutes

cooking: 4 to 5 minutes, plus 1 minute standing

Put the water in a large microwave-friendly bowl or storage container. Add the cauliflower and sprinkle the onion and dill on top. Lay a sheet of waxed paper on top of the bowl. Microwave on High until the cauliflower loses its raw taste and texture but is still crunchy, about 4 to 5 minutes. Let stand for 1 minute, then tip out any water accumulated in the bottom of the bowl. (Or, place the cauliflower florets in a steaming basket and sprinkle with the onion and dill. Steam over high heat until just tender, 3 to 5 minutes. Transfer to a bowl or storage container.)

Toss in the olive oil, lemon juice, salt, and pepper. Serve hot or at room temperature.

makes 4 side-dish servings

cauliflower and pasta salad: Cook and drain 4 to 6 ounces of shell-shaped pasta (tricolored is nice). Toss into the cauliflower salad. Add a few tablespoons each of drained capers and chopped drained sun-dried tomatoes. Splash on more lemon juice and olive oil and season to taste with more dill, salt, and freshly ground pepper.

southwest potato salad

2 pounds medium-sized red-skinned potatoes,
   scrubbed and quartered

1 teaspoon salt

2 cups fresh or frozen corn (use less if the salsa
   contains corn)

1 (15-ounce) jar tomato-based salsa

¼ to ½ cup chopped fresh cilantro (use less if the salsa contains cilantro)

1 jalapeño, seeded and minced (optional)

1 to 2 tablespoons plain or roasted garlic olive oil (optional)

Salt to taste

prep: 10 minutes
cooking: 12 to 15 minutes
cooling potatoes (optional): 15 to 30 minutes

Place the potatoes and salt in a large pot with ample water to cover. Bring to a boil, cover, and cook over medium heat until tender but still firm, 12 to 15 minutes. A minute or two before the potatoes are cooked, add the corn. Thoroughly drain the potatoes and corn. If time permits, allow the potatoes to cool before dicing them.

Dice the potatoes and place them, along with the corn, in a serving bowl or storage container. Stir in the salsa, cilantro, and jalapeño (if using), and adjust the seasoning as needed with olive oil and salt to taste. Serve warm or at room temperature.

makes 6 side-dish servings

cooking under pressure: Set the potatoes in a steaming basket over 1½ cups of water. Pressure-cook for 4 minutes under high pressure. Use a quick-release method. Remove the potatoes and steaming basket, and toss the fresh or frozen corn into the hot water. Cook, uncovered, until tender, about 1 minute. Drain and proceed with the recipe.

This spirited version of potato salad uses a zesty salsa dressing instead of mayonnaise. Splurge on the tastiest store-bought salsa available. If your salsa is fat-free, the salad is likely to need "smoothing out" with the addition of a tablespoon or two of plain or roasted garlic olive oil. For an indulgent touch, toss in a diced avocado.

Just-boiled potatoes are difficult to dice neatly so I usually let them cool first, but don't be concerned if you don't have time. Just use a knife and fork to cut them, and you'll have a slightly crumbly but still very delicious salad.

This salad tastes best when eaten within twenty-four hours.

coleslaw with creamy dill dressing

I love slaws and often serve one instead of a tossed salad—especially since it's so easy to store a sturdy green cabbage in the vegetable bin. In this recipe, the silken tofu does a terrific job standing in for the mayo, providing the appealing creaminess we associate with a traditional deli-style coleslaw. Substitute a few cups of red cabbage for the green, or toss in halved cherry tomatoes for an added splash of color if you like.

$\frac{1}{2}$ cup silken tofu ("lite" is fine)

1 small bunch fresh dill, tough stems removed (see page 8)

2 tablespoons mild white wine vinegar (not distilled!)

2 tablespoons freshly squeezed lemon juice

1 tablespoon olive oil

1 teaspoon salt, or to taste

$\frac{3}{4}$ pound green cabbage, shredded (6 to 7 loosely packed cups)

1 cup grated or finely chopped carrots

$\frac{1}{4}$ cup minced red onion

prep: 10 to 15 minutes

In a food processor or blender, process the tofu, dill, vinegar, lemon juice, oil, and salt until smooth. Place the cabbage, carrots, and onion in a large bowl or storage container, add the dressing, and toss to coat. Serve immediately or refrigerate for up to 4 days.

makes 6 servings

asian slaw

3 tablespoons brown rice or seasoned rice vinegar

2 tablespoons toasted sesame oil

Approximately 1½ tablespoons tamari

¾ pound Napa or green cabbage, shredded
(6 to 7 loosely packed cups)

1 cup grated or finely chopped carrots

1 cup thinly sliced scallion greens

¼ to ⅓ cup chopped fresh cilantro

Hot red pepper sauce, such as Tabasco, to taste (optional)

prep: 10 to 15 minutes

To make the dressing, in a large bowl or storage container, blend the vinegar, oil, and 1½ tablespoons tamari with a fork or a whisk. Add the cabbage, carrots, scallions, and cilantro, and toss well. Add extra tamari to taste and a few shakes of hot pepper sauce if you like. Serve immediately. Leftovers may be refrigerated for up to 4 days.

makes 6 servings

Slaw takes on a whole new personality when made with Napa cabbage and dressed with Asian condiments. Napa cabbage is delicate, however, and quickly loses its crunch once you add the dressing. If you will need to toss in the dressing more than a half hour in advance, substitute the sturdier green head cabbage.

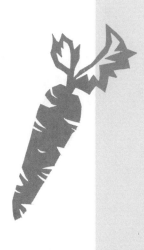

coleslaw with peanut sauce

Peanut sauce works wonders with raw cabbage, bringing richness to this humble vegetable and catapulting it to gourmet status. If you like, toss in a quarter cup of chopped fresh cilantro for additional Asian flavor.

**¾ pound green cabbage, shredded
(6 to 7 loosely packed cups)**

**1 cup finely chopped red bell peppers or
carrots**

½ cup thinly sliced scallion greens

⅓ to ½ cup Asian Peanut Sauce (page 22)

Tamari and/or seasoned rice vinegar to taste (optional)

prep: under 10 minutes
(assuming prepared sauce)

Place the cabbage, pepper, and scallions in a large bowl or storage container. Toss in enough sauce to coat thoroughly. Add tamari and/or a sprinkling of seasoned rice vinegar if you like, to make the flavors pop.

makes 4 servings

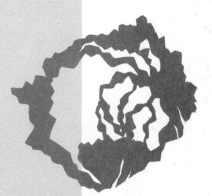

moroccan carrot slaw

2 tablespoons roasted garlic olive oil or

    2 tablespoons plain olive oil plus 1 to 2 small
    cloves garlic, minced

3 tablespoons freshly squeezed lemon juice

15 leafy sprigs fresh cilantro or parsley

1 teaspoon sweet Hungarian paprika

½ teaspoon ground cumin

½ teaspoon salt

4 to 5 large carrots, scrubbed or peeled and quartered

¼ cup dried currants

prep: about 10 minutes

In a food processor, blend the oil, lemon juice, cilantro, paprika, cumin, and salt until smooth. Pour the dressing into a large bowl or large storage container.

Add the carrots to the processor and pulse until finely chopped. (You should have about 4 cups.) Toss the carrots and currants in the dressing until well coated. Serve immediately, or cover and refrigerate for up to 3 days.

makes 4 servings

Slaws go beyond the realm of cabbage and can be created from chopped vegetables of all kinds. This carrot slaw is a personal favorite. It's good either freshly made or the next day, when the flavors have become more intense— almost pickled. The dried currants add a contrasting burst of color and sweetness.

For a light luncheon entrée, it's pleasant to serve this slaw over room-temperature basmati rice.

flash in the pan: hearty chilies, curries, stews, and stir-fries

The eclecticism of the American kitchen is perhaps no place more apparent than in this chapter, which includes chilies, curries, Thai-inspired stews, pasta fagioli, and stir-fries. As a nation of immigrants, we have long embraced the foreign as our own, so it feels quite natural to eat pasta one night and lo mein the next.

By the same token, our youthful spirit enables us to disregard long-hallowed culinary traditions and create new approaches to old favorites—approaches that accommodate formerly long-cooked stews to a short-cut lifestyle.

This is the chapter to turn to when you need a wholesome, flavor-packed meal in minutes. Each of the recipes makes use of one or more of the short-cut strategies I mentioned earlier, and they all add up to a new definition of fast food.

smoky black bean chili

Salsa gives this simple chili its instant soupy sauce. I've limited this bare-bones recipe to pantry ingredients so you can turn to it as a last-minute "what can we scare up for supper?" option. If you use top-notch store-bought salsa, it will be plenty good. (For a more plan-ahead, ingredient-packed chili, try the Bean and Corn Chili on page 88.)

I like to add a bit of oregano and chipotle chili powder to enhance the salsa's flavor and provide a hint of heat and smokiness. If you use a smoky salsa, however, you'll probably want to omit the chipotle (and Liquid Smoke). For heat without the smoke, use one-eighth teaspoon of cayenne.

Serve the chili in shallow bowls over pasta, rice, or instant polenta—perhaps with a few slices of avocado on top.

1¾ cups cooked black beans or
　1 (15-ounce) can black beans, drained
　(rinsed if nonorganic)
Approximately 1 cup store-bought tomato salsa
　(mild or hot, according to taste)
Scant ½ teaspoon dried oregano
⅛ teaspoon chipotle chili powder (see page 150)
　or approximately ¼ teaspoon Liquid Smoke
Salt to taste
1 tablespoon chopped fresh cilantro, for garnish (optional)

prep: about 5 minutes
cooking time: about 10 minutes

Combine beans, 1 cup salsa, the oregano, chili powder (if using Liquid Smoke, do not add it now), and salt in a medium saucepan. Bring to a boil, then reduce the heat and simmer, uncovered, until the beans take on a hint of the salsa's flavor, 7 to 10 minutes. Stir occasionally and add a bit more salsa or a few tablespoons of water if the chili becomes too dry.

Just before serving, stir in Liquid Smoke (if using) to taste. Garnish with cilantro (if you have happen to some around).

makes 2 servings

cook now, eat later

- Except for the stir-fries, all of the recipes in this chapter freeze beautifully. Make double or triple batches and freeze in microwavable portion sizes for future meals.
- Double stir-fry recipes and use leftovers for lunch, either on their own or stuffed into a pita pocket.
- To round out the meal, serve these saucy dishes over grains. Plan ahead by stocking your freezer with cooked whole grains (see page 34). Defrost and heat the amount you need.

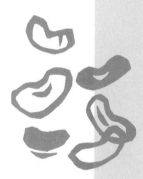

Here's a recipe to cook when you want a more serious chili than the quick smoky black bean version (page 86) but have neither the time nor the inclination to simmer a potful on the back of the stove. Despite this chili's short cooking time, the addition of lightly browned onions and garlic give it a longer-cooked taste. For more variety and visual appeal, use two different types of beans.

Unless you have a hot chili powder (sometimes called Mexican-style) you know and love, play it safe and use a mild blend. I like the Spice Garden brand available in many health food stores. You can always add a bit of Tabasco or cayenne at the end if you want the dish to be hotter.

For a change of pace, serve the chili over quinoa (see page 45). It's also great as a topping for a split-open baked potato.

bean and corn chili

1 tablespoon olive oil

1 medium onion, coarsely chopped

1 green or red bell pepper, cored, seeded, and diced

2 large cloves garlic, slivered

3½ cups cooked red kidney, black, or pinto beans or 2 (15-ounce) cans beans, drained (rinsed if nonorganic)

1 (14.5-ounce) can diced tomatoes with green chilies or Mexican-style stewed tomatoes with chipotles, coarsely chopped

1½ to 2 teaspoons mild chili powder

¼ teaspoon salt, or to taste

1½ cups fresh or frozen corn (no need to defrost)

⅓ cup chopped fresh cilantro

prep: about 10 minutes
cooking: about 10 minutes

In a large saucepan, heat the oil. Sauté the onion, bell pepper, and garlic over medium heat, stirring frequently, until lightly browned, 2 to 3 minutes. Add the beans, tomatoes, chili powder, and salt. Bring to a boil, then reduce the heat and simmer, uncovered, stirring occasionally, for 7 minutes.

Stir in the corn and continue cooking until the corn is tender, about 1 more minute. Stir in the cilantro and serve.

makes 4 servings

crunchy summer chili: Add 1 cup finely diced zucchini or jícama when you add the corn.

posole

1 (14.5-ounce) can diced tomatoes with
    green chilies or 1 (14.5-ounce) can
    Mexican-style stewed tomatoes with
    chipotles, coarsely chopped

1 (15-ounce) can white hominy (posole), drained and rinsed

1¾ cups cooked black, pinto, or red kidney beans or 1 (15-ounce) can
    beans, drained (rinsed if nonorganic)

1 cup fresh or frozen corn (no need to defrost)

1 teaspoon dried oregano

⅛ teaspoon chipotle chili powder (see page 150) or cayenne (optional)

Salt to taste

1 tablespoon roasted garlic olive oil

prep: 5 minutes
cooking: 5 minutes

In a large saucepan, combine all of the ingredients except the olive oil. Bring to a boil, then reduce the heat, partially cover, and simmer, stirring occasionally, until the flavors mingle and the ingredients are good and hot, about 5 minutes. Just before serving, stir in the olive oil.

makes 3 to 4 servings

I've named this bean-and-vegetable stew posole because it is based on the starchy, large-kernel corn that goes by that name in southwestern kitchens. In the East, posole is known as hominy. By any name, it has a delightfully chewy texture and subtle corn flavor. You'll find canned cooked hominy in most supermarkets (usually among the Goya products). It's quite salty, so be sure to rinse it well.

Set a bottle of Tabasco or other hot sauce on the table for those with asbestos tongues.

chickpea curry in a hurry

1 (14.5-ounce) can diced tomatoes
with green chilies or 1 (14.5-ounce)
can diced tomatoes plus 1 jalapeño, seeded
and diced

1 (10-ounce) package frozen chopped spinach

1¾ cups cooked chickpeas or 1 (15-ounce) can chickpeas, drained
(rinsed if nonorganic; reserve liquid if organic)

½ cup chickpea cooking liquid (if you have it), drained liquid from organic
canned beans, or water

1 tablespoon minced garlic

2 teaspoons Mild Curry Blend (page 17 or store-bought)

⅓ cup unsweetened, dried, grated coconut

½ teaspoon salt, or to taste

prep: 5 minutes
cooking: about 10 minutes

In a large saucepan, combine all the ingredients. Bring to a boil over high heat, then cover and cook over medium heat for 5 minutes. Break up the block of spinach with a fork, cover, and continue cooking until the spinach is cooked, about 5 more minutes. Stir well before serving.

makes 2 to 3 servings

chickpea curry soup: Thin leftover curry with vegetable stock and reheat. Stir in cooked basmati rice if you have some on hand.

This recipe is one of the crowning glories of my short-cut kitchen. Although it's a real "quick and easy" sort of dish, the curry tastes as if a great deal of time and effort went into the preparation. I suspect it will become a regular on your menu, and a standby to serve guests. (You can double or triple the recipe.)

Thanks for the success of this dish must go to a good-quality curry powder and the modest amount of dried coconut, which create a rich sauce that melds all of the ingredients together in a magical way. You can vary the taste by using different curry blends.

Serve the curry over boiled basmati rice with a dollop of your favorite chutney and perhaps some warm chapati—Indian flatbread—on the side.

bombay braised cabbage with tofu, peas, and corn

1 small head green cabbage (about 1 pound)

3 tablespoons tomato paste

1 cup warm water

1 tablespoon olive or canola oil

2 teaspoons black (brown) mustard seeds

1 teaspoon cumin seeds

2 teaspoons Mild Curry Blend (page 17 or store-bought)

1/2 teaspoon salt

1 pound firm tofu, drained and cut into 1/2-inch dice (see page 10)

1/2 cup frozen corn

1/2 cup frozen peas

2 to 3 tablespoons freshly squeezed lime juice

prep: under 10 minutes

cooking: 9 to 12 minutes

Cut the cabbage into 3-inch wedges and slice off any hard central core. Cut the wedges crosswise into slices about 1 inch thick. Set aside. In a cup, blend the tomato paste into the water.

Heat the oil in a large saucepan over high heat. Add the mustard and cumin seeds and let sizzle until the mustard seeds begin to pop, about 20 seconds. Immediately stir in the water–tomato paste mixture, curry, and salt. Add the cabbage and tofu and stir to coat with the sauce. Cover and cook over medium heat until the cabbage is just barely tender, about 8 minutes, stirring occasionally.

Add the corn and peas and continue cooking, covered, until the cabbage is wilted but still a bit crunchy, 1 to 3 more minutes. Just before serving, stir in lime juice to taste.

makes 3 servings

Cabbage and tofu really come alive when seasoned with Indian spices. I doubt that they've heard about this dish in Bombay, but I'd like to think they'd approve. Serve this curry over white or brown basmati rice. Or, cool to room temperature and sprinkle with additional lime juice to taste, and enjoy a Bombay cabbage salad.

orange-scented lentil ragout

Orange juice and zest plus a touch of cinnamon lend this otherwise earthy lentil-spinach ragout a fragrant, exotic note. You might want to double the recipe, since the mixture tastes even better after a short sojourn in the refrigerator.

Serve the stew in shallow bowls, either on its own or over basmati rice or bulgur. It also makes a nice topping for halved baked sweet potatoes or pasta spirals. If you're partial to parsley, this recipe works nicely with 1/4 cup minced fresh parsley in place of the spinach.

1 juice orange, preferably organic

1 tablespoon roasted garlic olive oil

1 cup thinly sliced leeks or coarsely chopped onions

1¾ cups cooked lentils or 1 (15-ounce) can lentils (plain or seasoned), drained (rinsed if nonorganic; reserve liquid if organic)

⅓ cup lentil cooking liquid (if you have it), drained liquid from organic canned beans, or water

1 (10-ounce) package frozen chopped spinach, defrosted (run under hot water in a sieve for a few minutes), or 1 (10-ounce) bag prewashed spinach, chopped

Scant ¼ teaspoon ground cinnamon, or to taste

Salt to taste

prep: about 10 minutes
cooking time: under 10 minutes

Using a peeler, remove half the orange zest and finely chop it. Cut the orange in half and squeeze out the juice. You should have about ⅓ cup. Set aside.

In a large saucepan, heat the oil and sauté the leeks for 1 minute, stirring frequently. Stir in the lentils, reserved cooking liquid, spinach, orange zest, cinnamon, and salt. Bring to a simmer, partially cover, and cook, stirring occasionally, until the leeks are cooked and the flavors have mingled, about 5 minutes. Just before serving, stir in the orange juice and add salt or cinnamon to taste if needed.

makes 3 to 4 servings

orange-scented lentil ragout with greens: Use chopped Swiss chard or beet greens instead of spinach.

pasta fagioli with cabbage

1 tablespoon olive oil

2 cups thinly sliced leeks or coarsely
   chopped onion

3 cups boiling water

1 tablespoon instant vegetable stock powder

2 teaspoons Italian Herb Blend (page 16 or store-bought)

1/2 cup small pasta, such as orzo, tubettini, or ditalini

1/2 pound green cabbage, coarsely chopped (about 4 loosely packed cups)

1 cup store-bought spaghetti sauce, preferably chunky-style with additions
   such as mushrooms and peppers

1¾ cups cooked chickpeas or 1 (15-ounce) can chickpeas, drained
   (rinsed if nonorganic)

Salt and freshly ground black pepper to taste

1/4 cup chopped fresh basil or parsley

1 to 3 teaspoons balsamic vinegar

1/4 cup grated Parmesan cheese (optional)

prep: about 10 minutes
cooking: under 15 minutes

In a large soup pot, heat the oil and sauté the leeks for 2 minutes, stirring frequently. Add the boiling water, stock powder, and herb blend and bring to a boil. Add the pasta and 2 cups of the cabbage. Cook at a rapid boil for 3 minutes less than the minimum time on the pasta package.

Stir in the pasta sauce, chickpeas, the remaining cabbage, and salt and pepper to taste and return to a boil. Reduce the heat to medium and cook, uncovered, stirring frequently (to prevent the pasta from sticking to the bottom of the pot), until the pasta is done, 3 to 4 more minutes.

Just before serving, stir in the basil and enough balsamic vinegar to sharpen the flavors. Add the Parmesan and more salt and pepper if needed.

makes 3 to 4 servings

Practically every cook in Italy makes her own version of pasta and beans. This is my short-cut version.

Since cabbage is always in my vegetable bin, one day I tossed some in along with the pasta and liked the result. My preference is to cook half of the cabbage until soft and add the remainder toward the end to give some crunch. However, you can add all of the cabbage at the beginning for a mellow texture.

The flavorful base is composed of three staples of the short-cut pantry: good-quality spaghetti sauce, Italian herb blend, and vegetable stock powder. And then there are those other two mainstays: pasta and cooked beans.

The stew thickens if refrigerated or left standing for a few hours. You can eat it that way or thin it by heating it with extra vegetable stock.

counting on cabbage

A while back, I began to notice how long cabbage lasts in the refrigerator—about ten days. While I'd gotten disgusted with having to throw away other tired, unused leafy greens and vegetables, cabbage was always ready, willing, and able. I began to depend upon it more and more for impromptu dinners and slaws.

Eventually, I got into the habit of keeping a head of green cabbage in the refrigerator at all times—occasionally supplementing it with a small head of red cabbage for color and variety. Ideas for recipes began to spring to mind (check the index to locate them), and I found myself going through my supply quite rapidly, using a large wedge here and half a head there.

Cabbage cooks very quickly and is adaptable to a wide range of seasonings and cooking techniques, so I actually find myself eating this healthy vegetable at least twice a week—or more, when I get a bad case of the munchies and a few slices of cabbage tossed with Annie's Sesame Shiitake Vinaigrette comes to the rescue.

It's quite easy to slice cabbage very thin using a serrated bread knife or the 2-mm. slicing disk of the food processor, but you can also buy the bagged, preshredded cabbage sold in supermarkets. Keep in mind, though, that it is more expensive and won't taste as fresh or last as long as the whole head.

cabbage and potatoes in mustard sauce

I tablespoon roasted garlic or plain olive oil

I cup thinly sliced leeks or coarsely chopped onions

I ½ cups water

Approximately I heaping tablespoon Dijon mustard

2 teaspoons instant vegetable stock powder

¼ to ½ teaspoon salt

¾ pound red-skinned potatoes, scrubbed and cut into I-inch cubes

I head green cabbage (about I pound)

Freshly ground black pepper to taste

prep: about 10 minutes
cooking: about 15 minutes

Heat the oil in a large saucepan over medium heat. Sauté the leeks for 1 minute, stirring frequently. Add the water and stir in 1 tablespoon mustard, the stock powder, and salt. Bring to a boil. Add the potatoes, cover, and cook for 5 minutes.

While the potatoes are cooking, cut the cabbage into wedges and slice off any hard core. Cut the wedges crosswise into slices about 1 inch thick.

Stir the cabbage into the potatoes. Add ⅓ cup of water if the mixture seems dry. Cover and cook over medium heat until the potatoes are fork-tender and the cabbage is tender with just a slight crunch, 9 to 12 minutes. Add a bit more mustard, if needed, and pepper to taste.

makes 3 servings

Dijon mustard lends its golden color to this homey combination of cabbage and potatoes, giving these two humble ingredients a touch of class and excellent flavor. If you like, add an herbaceous note with a heaping teaspoon of herbes de Provence (page 17 or store-bought), stirred in with the stock powder.

Serve over white or brown rice with a steamed green vegetable on the side.

Fortunately, many Southeast Asian ingredients that were formerly considered exotica are now found on supermarket shelves. You'll need Thai curry paste and a stalk of fresh lemon grass to get the great taste that this quick recipe delivers. If your supermarket doesn't carry them, try an Asian market. It's worth a bit of effort to have these ingredients on hand.

The incendiary curry paste comes in a jar or can and maintains its complex flavor indefinitely in the refrigerator. (Once it's been opened, transfer the paste from the can into a jar for long-term storage.) Unused stalks of lemon grass can be tightly wrapped in aluminum foil or a triple layer of plastic wrap and frozen for up to three months. (The flavor will diminish slightly.) Serve this memorable stew on its own or over Thai jasmine or Indian basmati rice.

thai-inspired red bean and sweet potato stew

1½ cups water

1 tablespoon instant vegetable stock powder

1 stalk lemon grass, outer bruised leaves removed, lower part only chopped into 2-inch pieces (discard grassy top)

1 teaspoon Thai red curry paste

1½ pounds sweet potatoes, peeled, quartered, and finely chopped (in a food processor)

1¾ cups cooked red kidney beans or 1 (15-ounce) can red kidney beans, drained (rinsed if nonorganic)

Salt to taste

prep: about 5 minutes
cooking: 10 minutes

In a large saucepan, combine the water, stock powder, lemon grass, and curry paste. Bring to a boil. Add the sweet potatoes, cover, and cook over medium heat for 7 minutes.

Stir in the kidney beans and salt to taste. Continue to cook, covered, until the sweet potatoes are very soft, about 3 more minutes. Add a bit more water if the mixture becomes too dry. Remove the pieces of lemon grass before serving.

makes 3 to 4 servings

broccoli stir-fry

⅓ cup water

¾ to 1 pound broccoli, trimmed and cut into
   florets and "coins" (stems sliced about
   ½ inch thick)

1 small red bell pepper, cored, seeded, and cut into thin strips

1 (8-ounce) can sliced water chestnuts, drained and rinsed

3 to 5 tablespoons Sesame-Ginger or Maple and Mustard Stir-Fry Sauce
   (page 25, or page 26, or store-bought)

⅛ to ¼ teaspoon crushed red pepper flakes (optional)

Tamari or shoyu to taste

prep: under 10 minutes
(assuming prepared
stir-fry sauce)

cooking: under 5 minutes

Bring the water to a boil in a wok or large skillet. Add the broccoli and bell pepper, cover, and cook over high heat until just short of done, about 2 minutes. Stir in the water chestnuts, 3 tablespoons stir-fry sauce, and the red pepper flakes (if using). Cook, stirring constantly, until the broccoli is crisp-tender, 1 to 2 more minutes. Taste and add extra stir-fry sauce and tamari if desired.

makes 2 servings

broccoli stir-fry with rice noodles: Cook 4 ounces of rice noodles as directed on the package; drain well. Add them to the stir-fry for the final minute, along with enough extra sauce to coat them thoroughly.

broccoli stir-fry with pasta: Use any leftover cooked pasta—spaghetti and fettuccine are especially nice—and proceed as directed in the variation above.

For a simple stir-fry, you can experiment with all sorts of dense vegetables, such as sliced Brussels sprouts or carrots, cauliflower florets, and, of course, broccoli. I've called for water chestnuts in the basic recipe, but you can stick exclusively with fresh vegetables or expand the dish by adding your favorite canned Chinese vegetables, such as bamboo shoots, baby corn, and straw mushrooms. (But do be sure to drain and rinse them thoroughly.) Just add extra stir-fry sauce at the end so all of the vegetables are well coated.

For a real short-cut, use frozen organic broccoli cuts (Cascadian Farms' are remarkably good) or the one-pound bag of stir-fry mixed vegetables found in supermarkets (not nearly as fresh tasting, but useful in emergencies). Cook the frozen vegetables the same way as described in the recipe.

baby corn with seasoned tofu and straw mushrooms

¼ to ⅓ cup **Sesame-Ginger or Maple and Mustard Stir-Fry Sauce (page 25, or page 26, or store-bought)**

1 tablespoon **minced fresh ginger (optional)**

1 pound **extra-firm tofu, drained and cut into ½-inch dice (see page 10)**

6 **scallions, cut into 2-inch pieces (keep the white and green parts separate; optional)**

1 (15-ounce) can **straw mushrooms, drained and rinsed**

1 (14.5-ounce) can **baby corn (sliced or whole), drained and rinsed**

prep: under 5 minutes (assuming prepared stir-fry sauce)

cooking: about 6 minutes

To make the seasoned tofu, in a wok or large skillet, combine ¼ cup stir-fry sauce, the ginger (if using), tofu, and scallion bulbs (if using). Bring to a boil, cover, and cook over medium heat for 4 minutes, stirring occasionally.

Toss in the straw mushrooms, corn, and scallion greens (if using) plus enough additional stir-fry sauce to coat the vegetables and give the dish a vibrant taste. Cover and cook over high heat until piping hot, 1 to 2 minutes.

makes 3 servings

cabbage, tofu, and red pepper stir-fry

3 to 4 tablespoons Sesame-Ginger
   or Maple and Mustard Stir-Fry Sauce
   (page 25, or page 26, or store-bought)

2 tablespoons water

1 pound green or Napa cabbage, very thinly sliced
   (7 to 8 loosely packed cups)

1 small red bell pepper, cored, seeded, and cut into thin strips

8 ounces baked seasoned tofu (such as White Wave Thai brand),
   cut into ½-inch dice

Tamari or shoyu to taste

prep: under 10 minutes
(assuming prepared stir-fry sauce)

cooking: about 6 minutes

In a wok or large skillet, mix 3 tablespoons stir-fry sauce with the water and bring to a boil over high heat. Add the cabbage and red pepper and stir to coat with the sauce. Toss in the tofu, cover, and continue to cook over high heat, stirring every minute or so, until the cabbage wilts but is still crunchy, 3 to 4 minutes (for Napa) or 4 to 6 minutes (for green). Stir in tamari to taste and add an additional tablespoon stir-fry sauce if desired.

makes 2 to 3 servings

This recipe calls for baked seasoned tofu, a flavorful firm tofu that is available in the refrigerator section of health food stores and Asian markets—or you can use the "homemade" seasoned tofu made from the previous recipe. If those alternatives aren't convenient, you can substitute plain extra-firm tofu and add a few extra tablespoons of stir-fry sauce. (The tofu won't have as much flavor, but its soothing blandness can actually be a nice contrast.)

The combination of cabbage and tofu makes a filling stir-fry that can stand on its own. For textural contrast and a more substantial meal, serve it over rice.

Here's a very pretty dish that is likely to become a real staple of your repertoire once you've gotten into the habit of having extra cooked grains on hand (see page 34). You can vary it with your favorite stir-fry sauce and expand on it as you wish. Here are some ideas:

- _With the grains, add small broccoli florets or carrots cut into quarter-inch-thick slices on the diagonal._
- _Include one or more types of canned Chinese vegetables, drained and rinsed, when you add the stir-fry sauce. Add extra sauce as needed to thoroughly coat all the ingredients._

whole-grain vegetable stir-fry

⅓ cup water

2 cups cooked whole grains (may be frozen)

1 large red bell pepper, cored, seeded, and
  cut into thin strips

3 scallions, thinly sliced (keep the white and green parts separate)

3 to 4 tablespoons Sesame-Ginger or Maple and Mustard Stir-Fry
  Sauce (page 25, or page 26, or store-bought)

½ cup frozen green peas or 3 ounces fresh snow peas, thinly sliced
  on the diagonal

Tamari to taste

prep: under 10 minutes
(assuming prepared stir-fry sauce)
cooking: about 5 minutes

In a wok or large skillet, bring the water to a boil. Add the grains, red pepper, and sliced scallion bulbs. Reduce the heat to medium and cook, covered, until the grains are tender and plump, about 2 minutes. Add 3 tablespoons stir-fry sauce, the peas, and scallion greens and cook, uncovered, for 2 minutes, stirring frequently.

Just before serving, stir in an additional tablespoon of stir-fry sauce if desired and add tamari to taste.

makes 2 servings

one-pot pasta
and grain entrées

When I ask busy people what they cook most often, the answer inevitably is pasta. I have a friend who makes dinner of pasta with store-bought pesto or tomato sauce two or three times a week. To amuse himself, he boils up different shapes and sizes, one night fusilli, another night linguine. While this strategy affords him a quick and delicious meal at home, I'm concerned that he has something of a mono-diet—and he certainly isn't eating enough fresh vegetables.

No one can deny that pasta is one of the most user-friendly foods around. But one of my aims in this chapter is to build more variety and nutrition into your pasta- and other grain-based suppers without costing you much extra time or effort.

sesame noodles with kale

1 large bunch kale (1¼ to 1½ pounds)

8 ounces udon, soba noodles, spaghetti, or fettuccine

1½ to 2 tablespoons toasted sesame oil

1½ to 2 tablespoons shoyu or tamari

1½ tablespoons toasted white or black sesame seeds

prep: under 10 minutes

cooking: 5 to 10 minutes
(depending upon type of pasta)

This and the following two recipes demonstrate a practical way to boil pasta and a green vegetable together to create a colorful entrée. I usually use brown-rice udon, which cooks in about the same amount of time it takes to tenderize kale—five minutes or so. If your pasta needs more cooking time than the vegetable, just give it a head start in the boiling water.

After draining the pasta and kale, save the cooking liquid to drink—piping hot and seasoned with a little tamari. (Or reserve the broth to enrich your next soup or vegetable stock.)

You'll start out with a huge mound of kale, but rest assured that greens shrink dramatically as they cook. Just be sure to use a very large pot.

While you are bringing a large pot of water to a boil, holding the bunch of kale together, slice off and discard the thickest part of the stems (about an inch or two). Still holding the kale in a bunch, slice the remaining stems and leaves as thin as you can. Set the kale in a sinkful (or large bowl) of water and swish vigorously to remove the grit. (Repeat this process with fresh water if the kale seems especially sandy.) Lift out the kale, place in a colander, and rinse thoroughly.

When the water has come to a rolling boil, add the pasta and cook it for 5 minutes less than the cooking time indicated on the package. Add the kale stems and leaves in a few batches, pressing down with the back of a large spoon to submerge each batch. Continue cooking, uncovered, over high heat until the kale and pasta are tender, about 5 more minutes. (The kale will tend to remain on top of the pasta. It's a good idea to press it under the water from time to time with the back of a large spoon.)

Drain the pasta and kale in a colander. (Bounce it up and down and tip side to side numerous times to release all the water caught in the kale's curly leaves.) Return the kale and pasta to the pot and toss in the toasted sesame oil and tamari to taste. With a fork, separate any kale leaves that have clumped together. Toss in the sesame seeds. Serve hot or at room temperature.

makes 3 servings

sesame noodle and kale salad: Add some chopped tomatoes, sliced scallions, or grated carrot, and an extra drizzle of sesame oil and tamari. Serve at room temperature.

more short-cuts to great grains and pastas
(see also "going with the grains," page 34)

- Experiment with pastas that are made partly of a whole grain, such as brown-rice udon or whole wheat spaghetti. Buy pasta made with organic flour if possible.
- Cook green vegetables along with the pasta, as I've done in the recipes on pages 102–105.
- Toss salad greens into just-cooked pasta (see page 106).
- Use an easy homemade vegetable-based sauce. For example, try spinach pesto (page 107) or Bean-Creamed Spinach (page 117).
- Expand your repertoire to include one-pot suppers based on other quick-cooking grains, such as instant barley, white rice, quinoa, and polenta.

Whenever I see a nice fresh bunch of broccoli rabe in the produce section, I can't resist making this simple dish. It's my favorite last-minute supper, and I never seem to tire of it.

Is it the slight bitter edge of the broccoli rabe or the crunchiness of the stems contrasted with the chewiness of the pasta? I'm not quite sure. (Look for perky greens, with no browning on the cut ends of the stems; avoid any bunches with yellowed or damaged leaves.)

Roasted garlic and basil olive oils marry remarkably well with soy sauce and offer tasty alternatives for the splash-on sauce—I often use a little of each. If I happen to have some imported black olives on hand, I toss some in. Leftovers are good at room temperature with a drizzle of lemon juice.

pasta with broccoli rabe and olives

1 good-sized bunch broccoli rabe
  (about 1¼ pounds)

8 ounces medium-sized pasta, such as
  penne, fusilli, or shells

⅓ cup pitted oil-cured olives

1 to 2 tablespoons roasted garlic, basil, or plain olive oil

1 to 2 tablespoons shoyu or tamari

Grated Parmesan cheese (optional)

prep: under 10 minutes
cooking: 5 to 10 minutes
(depending upon type of pasta)

While you are waiting for a large pot (six-quart or larger) of water to come to a boil, prepare the broccoli rabe: Discard any bruised or yellowed leaves. Holding the bunch together, trim off and discard the bottom 1 inch of the stems. Still holding it in a bunch, slice the remaining stems crosswise into 1-inch pieces. Place the stems in a colander, rinse, and set aside. Holding the greens in a bunch, cut the greens and florets (there won't be many) crosswise into about 1-inch pieces.

Cook the pasta in the rapidly boiling water for 4 minutes less than indicated on the package. Add the broccoli rabe stems and cook for 2 minutes. Meanwhile, place the leaves and florets in the empty colander and rinse.

Add the leaves and florets to the pasta (push them down to submerge them) and cook until the pasta is al dente, about 2 more minutes. Drain thoroughly. Return the pasta and broccoli rabe to the pot, or place in a serving bowl, and toss in the olives. Add the oil and shoyu to taste and toss again. Serve hot or at room temperature. Sprinkle with Parmesan if desired.

makes 2 to 3 servings

udon with green beans and peanut sauce

8 ounces brown-rice udon, rice noodles, or
    angel hair pasta

9 ounces frozen green beans, defrosted, or
    8 ounces fresh green beans, trimmed
    and cut into thirds

1/2 cup diced red or yellow bell pepper

1/3 to 1/2 cup **Asian Peanut Sauce (page 22)**

Tamari to taste (optional)

prep: 5 minutes
(assuming already-prepared
peanut sauce)

cooking: 5 to 10 minutes
(depending on type of pasta)

Bring a large pot of water to a rolling boil. Cook the pasta for 1 minute less than indicated on the package. Add the green beans and continue to cook until the pasta is done. Drain thoroughly in a colander, then transfer to a large bowl.

Toss in the red pepper and enough peanut sauce to coat. Add tamari to taste if desired. Serve warm or at room temperature.

makes 2 to 3 servings

udon with broccoli and peanut sauce: Use small broccoli florets or asparagus cut into 1-inch pieces instead of green beans. Add them to the boiling water 2 minutes before the pasta is done.

udon with snow peas and peanut sauce: Use 4 ounces of trimmed and stringed snow peas instead of the beans. Add them to the boiling water about a minute before the pasta is done.

udon with carrots, peas, and peanut sauce: Add 2 medium carrots, trimmed, peeled, and thinly sliced on the diagonal, 3 minutes before the pasta is done. One minute later, add 3/4 cup defrosted frozen peas.

Peanut sauce on noodles always seems luxurious and celebratory, perhaps because it reminds me of my favorite Chinese cold sesame noodles. My version is more temperate on the fat grams. I've also added a healthy portion of green beans and red peppers for a boost of nutrition and bright color.

To simplify preparation, the green beans are cooked along with the pasta. The timing given here yields crunchy beans. If you prefer tender beans, or if you're using fresh rather than frozen, add the beans a minute earlier than directed.

This dish is filling and makes a good one-pot supper. To make it heartier still, toss four to six ounces of diced seasoned baked tofu (available in the refrigerated and/or salad bar sections of most health food stores) into the cooked noodles.

Here's a nice way to have your pasta and salad all in one course! I was inspired to create this combination by the easy accessibility of top-notch mesclun. The mixed greens are stirred into the hot pasta, causing the leaves to wilt slightly. The result is a colorful and very tasty dish that offers intriguing variations in texture. Sometimes I'll heighten the drama even further by tossing in a few tablespoons of toasted pine nuts or about half a cup of diced red or yellow bell pepper.

To prevent the dish from becoming waterlogged, it's important to dry rinsed greens thoroughly in a salad spinner. (If you buy prewashed mesclun, you'll be all set.) Roasted garlic olive oil combined with tamari soy sauce again comes to the rescue for a remarkably good splash-on dressing.

pasta with wilted mesclun

8 ounces medium-sized pasta, such as
    fusilli, shells, or penne

6 ounces mesclun (or an equivalent amount
    of radicchio and watercress or arugula leaves,
    rinsed, trimmed, and chopped)

2 tablespoons roasted garlic olive oil

1 to 2 tablespoons tamari

Freshly ground black pepper to taste

Grated Parmesan cheese (optional)

prep: under 5 minutes
cooking: 5 to 10 minutes
(depending upon type of pasta)

Bring a large pot of water to a rolling boil. Add the pasta and cook according to the package directions until al dente. Drain thoroughly.

Return the pasta to the pot (or transfer to a heated serving bowl) and stir in the mesclun, oil, and tamari to taste. Continue to stir until the greens have wilted slightly. Season with black pepper to taste. Serve hot or at room temperature, with a sprinkling of Parmesan cheese if desired.

makes 2 to 3 servings

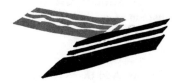

fettuccine with spinach pesto

8 ounces fettuccine

1 (10-ounce) package frozen spinach, defrosted

2 heaping tablespoons walnut halves

1 tablespoon freshly squeezed lemon juice, or more to taste, or 1 to 3 teaspoons balsamic vinegar

1 tablespoon basil (my preference) or roasted garlic olive oil, or a combination

1 teaspoon Italian Herb Blend (page 16 or store-bought)

1 small clove garlic (optional if using roasted garlic oil)

1/2 teaspoon salt, or to taste

Freshly ground black pepper to taste

Grated Parmesan cheese (optional)

prep: under 10 minutes
cooking: 5 to 12 minutes
(depending upon type of pasta)

Bring a large pot of water to a rolling boil. Cook the fettuccine according to the package directions until al dente.

Meanwhile, place the remaining ingredients except the Parmesan in a food processor and blend for about 30 seconds to create a coarse paste, scraping down the sides of the bowl as necessary.

When the pasta is done, drain it thoroughly. Place the pesto in the hot pot, add the pasta, and toss well. Add additional salt, pepper, and or lemon juice if needed, to make the flavors pop. Reheat if necessary. Garnish individual portions with a dusting of Parmesan if you like.

makes 2 servings

fettuccine with tomatoes, capers, and spinach pesto: Toss the pasta and pesto with 1 1/2 cups diced plum tomatoes and 1 to 2 tablespoons drained capers.

Our old reliable Italian herb blend and infused oils add an interesting herbal backdrop to this verdant low-fat pesto. By using frozen spinach rather than basil, you can make pesto on the spur of the moment, regardless of the season. Vary the dish by using spaghetti or shells instead of fettuccine.

I normally squeeze the excess liquid out of defrosted spinach, but in this recipe it's needed to thin the pesto. When defrosting the spinach (the microwave oven does the quickest job), set it on a plate to catch all of the liquid—or defrost it right in the bowl of your food processor (without the metal blade, if you're microwaving it). You'll have plenty of time to make the pesto while the water comes to a boil and the pasta cooks.

red-hot black beans and rice

2 cups water

2 tablespoons tomato paste

I tablespoon instant vegetable stock powder

I tablespoon roasted garlic olive oil or I tablespoon plain olive oil
   plus I teaspoon minced garlic

I teaspoon dried oregano

I teaspoon cumin seeds

¼ teaspoon salt, or to taste

¼ to ½ teaspoon crushed red pepper flakes (use the larger amount
   if you like your food really hot)

I cup extra-long-grain white rice

½ cup coarsely chopped pimento-stuffed green olives

1¾ cups cooked black beans or I (15-ounce) can black beans, drained
   (rinsed if nonorganic)

½ cup thinly sliced scallion greens

prep: under 10 minutes

cooking: about 20 minutes,
plus 2 minutes standing

From India to Mexico to New Orleans, rice and beans show up in many of the world's kitchens, and for good reason: It's an economical duo that nourishes both body and soul.

You won't need to add much salt to this Caribbean-inspired recipe since the olives season the rice as the mixture cooks. A drizzle of lime juice perks up leftovers to make a tasty room-temperature salad.

In a large saucepan, combine the water, tomato paste, stock powder, oil, oregano, cumin, salt, and red pepper flakes and bring to a boil over high heat. Stir in the rice and olives. Return to a boil, then cover, lower the heat, and simmer for 18 minutes.

Quickly scatter the beans on over the rice. Cover and remove from the heat. Let sit until the rice is tender and beans are thoroughly heated, about 2 minutes. Stir in the scallions, distributing the beans as you fluff up the rice.

makes 3 servings

paella vegetariana

1 tablespoon olive oil

1 cup thinly sliced leeks or coarsely
  chopped onions

1½ teaspoons minced garlic

2¼ cups water

1 tablespoon instant stock powder

½ teaspoon saffron threads

½ to ¾ teaspoon salt, or to taste

1¼ cups extra-long-grain white rice

1 cup diced carrots

1 cup frozen peas, defrosted, or 1½ cups sliced defrosted artichoke hearts

1 cup frozen corn, defrosted

1¾ cups cooked red kidney beans or 1 (15-ounce) can red kidney beans,
  drained (rinsed if nonorganic)

½ cup diced roasted red pepper (page 9 or store-bought)

Freshly ground black pepper to taste

¼ cup toasted sliced almonds, for garnish (optional)

prep: about 10 minutes

cooking: about 20 minutes,
plus 2 minutes standing

Heat the oil in a large heavy saucepan. Sauté the leeks and garlic over medium heat for 1 minute, stirring frequently. Stir in the water, stock powder, saffron, and salt, rubbing the saffron between your fingers to release its flavor as you add it. Bring to a boil. Stir in the rice and carrots. Cover, reduce the heat, and simmer for 18 minutes.

Quickly sprinkle the peas, corn, kidney beans, and red pepper on top of the rice. Cover and remove from the heat. Let sit until the rice is tender and the vegetables are thoroughly heated, about 2 minutes. Add pepper to taste and additional salt if needed. Stir well. Transfer to a serving bowl and sprinkle with the almonds (if using).

makes 4 servings

Picture perfect—with its saffron-golden rice, mahogany kidney beans, and bright green peas—this elegant vegetarian version of paella is a great dish to serve company. Don't feel daunted by the length of the ingredients list, because the dish is actually very easy to assemble.

Using leeks instead of onions gives the dish a memorable flavor boost. A green salad tossed with Very Versatile Vinaigrette (page 19) makes a good accompaniment to the paella.

Combining Asian ginger, tamari, and aduki beans with quinoa and squash from the Americas is a good example of the kind of fusion cooking that makes eating an exciting adventure.

If you need some instructions on preparing the squash, see page 10. It's important to cut it into small pieces so that it will be tender by the time the quinoa is done.

gingered quinoa with butternut squash and beans

1½ cups water

1 tablespoon tamari, or more to taste

1 cup quinoa, thoroughly rinsed and drained
   (see page 45)

1 piece fresh ginger, about 1 inch square, peeled and finely minced

1 large clove garlic, finely minced

½ to ¾ pound butternut squash, peeled, seeded, and cut into ½-inch dice
   (about 3 cups)

1¾ cups cooked aduki beans, heated, or 1 (15-ounce) can Eden Foods
   organic aduki or gingered black beans, heated and drained (see Note)

½ cup thinly sliced scallion greens

prep: about 15 minutes

cooking: 12 to 15 minutes

In a medium saucepan, bring the water and tamari to a boil. Add the quinoa, ginger, garlic, and squash. Return to a boil, then reduce heat to medium and cook, covered, until the quinoa and squash are tender and the liquid is absorbed, 12 to 15 minutes. If all the liquid is absorbed and the quinoa is not yet tender, stir in 2 to 3 tablespoons of boiling water, cover, and simmer until done. (Alternatively, if the quinoa and squash are tender and there is still liquid left in the pot, drain it off and return the mixture to the pot.)

Toss in the heated beans and scallions as you fluff up the quinoa. Season with additional tamari if desired.

note: If you have trouble finding these, substitute black soybeans or regular black (turtle) beans.

makes 3 to 4 servings

tex-mex quinoa pilaf with potatoes and corn

1½ cups water

1 tablespoon instant vegetable stock powder

1 cup quinoa, thoroughly rinsed and drained (see page 45)

¾ pound thin-skinned potatoes, scrubbed and cut into ½-inch dice
   (about 3 cups)

1 teaspoon cumin seeds

½ teaspoon salt, or more to taste

1 cup frozen corn, defrosted

½ cup diced roasted red pepper (page 9 or store-bought)

¼ cup chopped fresh cilantro or parsley or scallion greens

prep: under 15 minutes

cooking: 12 to 15 minutes

In a medium heavy saucepan, bring the water and stock powder to a boil over high heat. Stir in the quinoa, potatoes, cumin, and salt, cover, and simmer over low heat for 10 minutes.

Add the corn and continue cooking until the quinoa and potatoes are tender and all the liquid is absorbed, 12 to 15 minutes. If all the liquid is absorbed and the quinoa is not yet tender, stir in 2 to 3 tablespoons of boiling water, cover, and continue simmering until done. (Alternatively, if the quinoa and potatoes are tender and there is still liquid left in the pot, drain it off.)

Season with additional salt if needed, and stir in the red pepper and cilantro.

makes 2 to 3 servings

tex-mex quinoa soup: Stir leftovers into a pot of vegetable stock (allow 1 heaping teaspoon instant stock powder per cup of boiling water). Liven up with a squeeze of lime.

I'm convinced that quinoa will become the rice of the nineties, as more and more people discover this light, quick-cooking, nutritious grain.

It's only natural that quinoa, potatoes, and corn go so well together: They are all indigenous to Latin America. However, here the success of this delicious combination depends upon cutting the potatoes properly—if they are larger than half-inch cubes, they will not be tender when the quinoa is done.

Accompany the pilaf with a salad or steamed green vegetable for a terrific meal.

Plain polenta can be the best comfort food in the world, but there are times when I'm feeling extravagant and want to gussy it up. With this in mind, there's nothing simpler or better than stirring in an abundance of crunchy artichoke hearts. A spoonful of spaghetti sauce on top completes the treat. Or, when I'm in a South-of-the-border mood, I pour on salsa instead.

Whatever you do, serve the polenta piping hot, immediately after it's cooked; it firms up quickly as it cools.

polenta with artichoke hearts

2¼ cups water

1 teaspoon Italian Herb Blend
(page 16 or store-bought)

½ teaspoon salt

1 (9-ounce) package frozen artichoke hearts

½ cup quick-cooking polenta

2 tablespoons grated Parmesan cheese (optional)

1 tablespoon drained capers (optional)

1 tablespoon roasted garlic olive oil

Lots of freshly ground black pepper

¾ cup store-bought spaghetti sauce, heated

prep: 5 minutes

cooking: about 8 minutes

In a medium saucepan, bring the water, herbs, and salt to a boil. Add the artichoke hearts and return to a boil. Cover, lower the heat to medium, and cook until the artichokes are just short of tender, 4 to 5 minutes. (I like the artichoke hearts big and chunky, but you may prefer to lift them out with a slotted spoon and slice them, then return them to the water.)

While stirring constantly with a fork, gradually sprinkle in the polenta. Cook, uncovered, at a gentle boil, stirring constantly, until the polenta thickens, 1 to 2 minutes. Stir in the Parmesan cheese and capers (if using), oil, and pepper. Serve in shallow bowls with the hot spaghetti sauce on top.

makes 2 servings

vegetables à la carte

As you probably have noticed, I've made a sustained effort to tuck vegetables into practically every recipe in this book. And, in truth, I eat most of my vegetables incorporated into soups, stews, salads, and pasta dishes.

However, there are times when it's nice to single out a particular vegetable or two and give them special attention. On those occasions when I do so, I often feel as though I've given myself a special treat.

A case in point is Gingery Steamed Kabocha Squash. Often when I see a kabocha squash in the natural food store, I have an inner dialogue about whether or not I feel like taking the time to chop the thing up. (It does require a sharp chef's knife and considerable elbow grease.) But if I decide to bring one home, I rarely wait more than a day to steam it as described on page 126. Then the inner voice goes something like this: "Even better than I remembered. I should really do this more often."

The same is true for baked potatoes. Is there anything more satisfying than a crispy-skinned one, split open and steaming hot? While it's baking, the kitchen smells as good as homemade bread. But months could go by between one baked potato and the next. That is, until I came up with the strategy of popping a few russets into the oven anytime I had it turned on, so that I often have baked potatoes on hand, ready to be reheated (see page 123).

In this chapter, I've suggested a number of approaches that make it easy and fun to give some terrific vegetables the attention they deserve. I've also shown you numerous ways to turn a simple vegetable into a whole meal.

roasted portobello mushrooms

2 large portobello mushrooms
   (about 4 ounces each, with caps
   measuring approximately
   4½ inches across)
1 tablespoon roasted garlic olive oil
Salt to taste

prep: 5 minutes
roasting: 10 minutes

Position the rack in the center of the oven and preheat the oven to 450 degrees.

Trim off the earthy root ends and lightly wipe the portobello caps and stems with a damp cloth. Leave the gills intact. Slice off the stems and cut them lengthwise into ½-inch-thick slices.

Set the mushroom caps gill side up in a shallow ovenproof baking dish just large enough to hold them and lightly brush with half the oil. Season with salt to taste, turn them over, and brush with the remaining oil. Roast, uncovered, for 5 minutes. Flip over and scatter the sliced stems between the caps. Roast until the mushrooms are just tender, about 5 more minutes.

Serve the caps whole, or slice each one on the bias (by holding the knife at a slant) to create about six or seven "fingers." Scatter the stems on top.

makes 2 servings

portobello mashed potatoes: Chop any leftover roasted portobellos and stir them into mashed potatoes. What a treat!

I regret how long it took me to discover portobello mushrooms. I'm not sure what held me back, but if you've been as sluggish as I, please don't wait a moment longer.

Succulent and juicy, portobellos are the "steak" of the vegetable kingdom. The simple act of roasting them for ten minutes intensifies their earthy flavor and sears in their abundant juices. Slice the caps into "fingers" and fan them out over a mound of Basic Polenta scented with rosemary (page 37). Surround the polenta with mesclun tossed in Very Versatile Vinaigrette (page 19), and garnish with the chopped mushroom stems for a royal feast.

roasted parsnip spears

I pound slender parsnips, peeled, trimmed, and halved lengthwise

I tablespoon plain or rosemary olive oil

prep: 5 minutes
roasting: 25 minutes

Place the oven rack in the bottom third of the oven and preheat the oven to 450 degrees.

In a large shallow baking dish, toss the parsnips in the oil. Arrange cut side down, preferably in one layer, and roast, uncovered, for 15 minutes. Use tongs to flip over, and roast until the parsnips are easily pierced with a paring knife, about 10 minutes longer.

makes 2 to 4 servings

bean-creamed spinach

1 tablespoon olive oil

1 cup coarsely chopped onions

1¾ cups cooked navy or cannellini beans or 1 (15-ounce) can
    navy or cannellini beans, drained (rinsed if nonorganic)

1 (10-ounce) package frozen spinach

1 cup water

1 tablespoon instant vegetable stock powder

2 teaspoons dried dill or ⅛ teaspoon freshly grated nutmeg

½ teaspoon salt, or to taste

2 tablespoons freshly squeezed lemon juice (optional)

Freshly ground black pepper to taste

prep: under 10 minutes

cooking: 10 minutes

Heat the oil in a medium saucepan. Sauté the onions for 1 minute, stirring frequently. Add the beans, spinach, water, stock powder, dill, and salt and bring to a boil over high heat. Cover and cook over medium heat for 5 minutes.

Break up the block of spinach with a fork and stir well. Cook until the spinach is tender, 3 to 5 minutes. Puree the mixture with an immersion blender (or transfer in small batches to a food processor or blender and puree until smooth).

If the creamed spinach seems too thick, thin slightly with lemon juice, which will sharpen the flavors, or with water. Season with pepper to taste. Depending upon the consistency, serve either in small bowls or on plates.

makes 4 servings

In this remarkably tasty side-dish vegetable, instant stock powder provides a long-cooked depth of flavor in minutes. The rich creaminess of the white beans transforms frozen spinach into a healthful and delicious version of creamed spinach.

It's not just a side dish though: Use leftover "creamed" spinach as a sauce for pasta or grains (season a bit more heavily) or thin it with enough vegetable stock to turn it into a soup.

A bunch of fresh young tender spinach with the roots still attached is a real treasure. It requires careful dunking to rinse off any grit—which can seem like a nuisance—but you are rewarded with an intensely flavored vegetable, roots and all. (Why were we ever taught to toss them away?) Of course, if you're pressed for time, prewashed spinach is a good option.

Microwaved spinach has such intense flavor that I prefer to eat it plain. If you like, however, sprinkle on some herbed seasoning salt (Herbamare is a personal favorite) or lightly glaze the leaves with toasted sesame oil and tamari.

intense micro spinach

8 to 10 ounces spinach

Herbed seasoning salt to taste (optional)

prep: about 5 minutes
cooking: 4 minutes,
plus 1 minute standing

Wash the spinach by swishing it gently but persistently in a sinkful (or large bowlful) of cold water. Lift out of the water, leaving the grit behind. Repeat if the spinach still seems sandy. Coarsely chop the spinach and roots, trimming off any browned parts. Place in a colander to drain slightly.

Place the spinach in a large microwave-friendly bowl, with the rinsing water still clinging to the leaves. Lay a sheet of waxed paper on top of the bowl. Microwave on High for 4 minutes; let stand for 1 minute. Tip out any water accumulated in the bottom of the bowl or, with a slotted spoon, transfer the spinach to a smaller bowl. Sprinkle with seasoning salt if you wish.

makes 2 servings

microwave magic

Like many cooks, I use my microwave primarily to reheat and defrost foods. However, I have discovered how well it cooks certain vegetables—fresh kale, spinach, and cauliflower, to be precise. Thanks to the microwave, I now eat these fresh vegetables more regularly and really enjoy their excellent color, texture, and taste. You'll find a few of my favorite microwave vegetable recipes scattered throughout this chapter—plus a tasty Dilled Cauliflower Salad on page 78. All recipes were tested in an 850-watt oven on High (100%) power.

micro kale

8 ounces kale

Freshly squeezed lemon juice and olive oil or tamari and toasted sesame oil (optional)

prep: about 5 minutes
cooking: about 4 minutes, plus 1 minute standing

Holding the kale together in a bunch, cut off the stems about 3 inches below the leaves and discard. Still holding the kale in a bunch, slice the remaining stems and leaves about ¼ inch thick. Swish the kale vigorously in a sinkful (or large bowlful) of water to remove the grit. (Repeat this process with fresh water if the kale seems especially sandy.) Lift out the kale, place in a colander, and rinse thoroughly.

Place the kale in a large microwave-friendly bowl, with its rinsing water still clinging to the leaves. Lay a sheet of waxed paper on top of the bowl. Microwave on High for 4 minutes. Let stand 1 minute, then taste, and if the kale is not sufficiently tender, microwave for 30 to 60 seconds longer. Tip out any water accumulated in the bottom of the bowl or, with a slotted spoon, transfer the kale to a smaller bowl.

Toss with a splash of lemon juice and olive oil or toasted sesame oil and tamari if you wish.

makes 2 servings

single serving: It's quite a boon to be able to prepare single quantities of this delicious vegetable so easily. Halve the recipe to 4 ounces of kale and reduce the cooking time to 3 minutes to yield 1 cup cooked kale.

Microwaving preserves kale's bright green color and intensifies its taste. I usually eat the kale right from the cooking bowl, with perhaps a light coating of olive oil and lemon juice or toasted sesame oil and tamari. (I never add salt or pepper, as I find kale flavorful enough without them.) I'll often eat "micro kale" on a heap of Fluffy Smashed Potatoes (page 124), as one of my most reliable quick meals. It's also delicious on top of a bed of grains, coated with Asian Peanut Sauce (page 22).

A half pound of fresh kale (about eight cups chopped) shrinks to about two cups cooked—a good-sized portion for two. The best time to microwave kale is when you find young tender (usually small) leaves with thin stems. Older kale is more effectively tenderized by boiling or steaming.

spinach with toasted coconut and black mustard seeds

This is one of the best ways I've discovered for preparing spinach. I'm enchanted with the flavor of toasted black mustard seeds, and coconut runs a close second on my roster of preferred ingredients—so why not combine the two, as Indian cooks have done for millennia? The coconut gives the spinach a touch of class and the mustard seeds add a spicy crunch.

When using a bunch of fresh young spinach that has the delicate pink roots still intact, cook the roots along with the spinach for a special treat. (Just rinse them well to remove any dirt and trim off any brown parts; see instructions on page 10.)

For a nice dinner triad, serve the spinach with basmati rice and Thai-Inspired Red Bean and Sweet Potato Stew (page 96).

1 teaspoon safflower or canola oil

3 tablespoons unsweetened dried grated coconut

2 teaspoons black (brown) mustard seeds

1¼ pounds spinach, trimmed, thoroughly washed, and coarsely chopped, or 2 (10-ounce) bags prewashed spinach

¼ to ½ teaspoon salt

prep: about 5 minutes
cooking: 4 minutes

In a large nonstick saucepan or large wok, heat the oil over high heat. Toast the coconut and mustard seeds, stirring constantly, until the coconut turns light brown and the seeds pop like crazy, about 30 seconds.

Add the spinach, with the water still clinging to the leaves (if using prewashed spinach, sprinkle on 3 tablespoons of water), and the salt. Cook, uncovered, over medium-high heat, stirring frequently, until the spinach is tender, about 3 minutes. Lift from the pan with a slotted spoon.

makes 4 servings

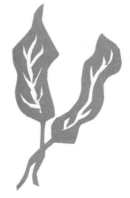

steamed new potatoes with lemon-garlic sauce

1 pound small new potatoes, scrubbed
   and halved

2 tablespoons freshly squeezed lemon juice

1 tablespoon roasted garlic olive oil

1 teaspoon Dijon mustard

1/8 teaspoon salt

Freshly ground black pepper to taste

3 tablespoons minced fresh parsley, for garnish (optional)

prep: under 5 minutes
cooking: about 15 minutes

Pour 2 cups of water into a large saucepan fitted with a collapsible vegetable steamer, and fill the steamer with the halved potatoes. Bring the water to a boil over high heat, then cover and cook over medium-high heat until the potatoes are tender, about 15 minutes.

Meanwhile, in a medium bowl, blend the remaining ingredients (except the parsley) with a small whisk or a fork.

Add the hot potatoes to the sauce and toss. Garnish with the parsley if you wish, and serve hot or at room temperature.

makes 2 to 3 servings

To add instant pizzazz to boiled new potatoes (or steamed or microwaved green vegetables), try this quick sauce. Change the personality of the sauce by using your favorite flavored mustard—honey, horseradish, peppercorn, or tarragon, to name a few.

To keep cleanup to a minimum, combine the sauce ingredients in a serving bowl while the potatoes are steaming.

Keep a few aseptic packages of silken tofu in your cupboard to make last-minute potato toppings like this cholesterol-free alternative to butter and sour cream. The topping also works as a vegetable dip, or it can be turned into a mayo-like spread for sandwiches filled with grilled vegetables.

The amount of horseradish you'll need will vary according to its potency—the sharpness fades with age—and your love of its flavor.

(Use the tofu left over from a ten-ounce package to make the Creamy Dill Dressing on page 80.)

baked potatoes with zesty tofu topping

5 ounces (half of a 10-ounce aseptic pack) regular or "lite" silken tofu

2 tablespoons catsup or store-bought tomato sauce

1 tablespoon prepared red or white horseradish, or more to taste

1 tablespoon Dijon mustard

1 scallion, cut into 4 pieces, or 1 tablespoon freeze-dried chives

1/2 teaspoon salt

3 baked potatoes, heated and split

prep: 5 minutes (assuming already-baked potatoes)

In a food processor, combine all of the ingredients except the potatoes and process to a smooth puree. Taste and add more horseradish as desired. (The topping can be prepared up to 5 days ahead, covered, and refrigerated. Bring to room temperature and stir well before using.)

Serve the topping spooned over the hot baked potatoes.

makes 3 servings

thoughts on baked potatoes

Baked potatoes hardly qualify as a quick fix. Microwaving potatoes works in emergencies, but the soft skins and inner texture of microwaved potatoes really don't satisfy that deep inner yearning. Because of my love of crispy potato skins and the texture unique to oven-baked potatoes, I got into the habit of setting a few directly on an oven rack to bake along with whatever I'm making at the time. Although the potatoes are best when freshly baked, I refrigerate extras for up to five days and reheat (and recrisp) them in the toaster oven.

Look for long, skinny russet (Idaho) potatoes, since the thin ones bake faster than chubby specimens and are done in about thirty-five to forty minutes at 375 to 425 degrees. Don't worry about being particularly specific with the oven temperature. The potatoes will do fine anywhere in that fifty-degree range.

For a quick and hearty entrée, reheat the baked potatoes in a toaster oven or microwave, slit them open, and top each half with some warmed-up canned or homemade chili, baked beans, or seasoned lentils. Sprinkle some minced parsley or cilantro on top if you like.

For an enjoyable light lunch or snack, try a baked potato, halved and coarsely mashed with cottage cheese or soy yogurt, thinly sliced scallions, a sprinkling of herb seasoning salt (such as Herbamare), and freshly ground black pepper. Or whip up a batch of Zesty Tofu Topping (page 122) and top the potato with a dollop or two.

Here's a quick, down-home, low-fat version of mashed potatoes that I prepare in the microwave. I don't peel the potatoes, since the skin has such good flavor. If you prefer a creamier version, add a tablespoon or two of water while you are smashing the potatoes.

Served plain, these fluffy potatoes make a great cushion for chili and other bean stews. But I've been known to eat one for my entire dinner, gussied up with one or more add-ons, and accompanied by thinly sliced cabbage tossed with a splash-on dressing of olive oil and lemon juice.

fluffy smashed potatoes

¼ cup water

2 large russet potatoes (about 8 ounces each), scrubbed or peeled and cut into eighths

3 to 4 large cloves garlic (optional)

Salt and freshly ground black pepper to taste

Optional add-ons:

    thinly sliced scallions

    chopped fresh parsley, dill, or basil

    1 to 2 tablespoons roasted garlic, rosemary, or basil olive oil

    1 to 2 tablespoons Dijon mustard

    ¼ to ½ cup chopped leftover steamed vegetables

prep: under 10 minutes

cooking: 7 to 10 minutes, plus 1 minute standing

Place the water, potatoes, and garlic (if using) in a medium microwave-friendly bowl. Lay a sheet of waxed paper on top of the bowl. Microwave on High until the potatoes are fork-tender, 7 to 10 minutes. Let stand for 1 minute.

Use a potato masher or fork to coarsely smash the potatoes, adding a few tablespoons of water if the mixture seems dry. Season to taste with salt and pepper, and with any of the add-ons that strike your fancy.

makes 2 to 3 servings

elizabeth's steamed sweets

2 medium sweet potatoes (about 8 ounces
    each), preferably long and thin, scrubbed
    and cut lengthwise in half

prep: 1 to 2 minutes
cooking: 12 to 15 minutes

Pour about 2 cups of water in a large saucepan and set a steamer basket in place. Arrange the sweet potatoes, cut side up, in the basket. Cover the pot and bring the water to a boil over high heat, then cook over medium-high heat until the potatoes are fork-tender, 12 to 15 minutes. Serve as is, or scoop the flesh out of the skins and cut into chunks, or mash.

note: These instructions are for cooking 2 sweet potatoes, but make as many as you like by stacking the potatoes pyramid-fashion in the vegetable steamer.

makes 2 servings

A dear friend and esteemed colleague, produce specialist Elizabeth Schneider, alerted me to this delicious and efficient way to cook sweet potatoes. I'd always baked sweet potatoes and was surprised to find that steaming brings out their good flavor and creaminess in about a third the time.

To minimize cooking time, select the skinniest potatoes available. Certain varieties, if you can find them, are naturally elongated. Personal favorites are the Jewel variety and garnet yams, available at many natural food stores and some farmers' markets.

Recently I made a terrific meal by setting chunks of peeled steamed sweets over rice, and topping the mound with warmed Asian Peanut Sauce (page 22). Wow!

When you come across a full-flavored, densely textured squash such as kabocha or delicata—almost always available in health food stores that carry produce—make this recipe for an intense squash experience. If the squash is organic, you won't have to peel the edible skin, which is a great timesaver—and it looks pretty too.

To avoid scorching the squash on the bottom of the pot, check frequently toward the end of the cooking time to see if you need to add a bit more water. (I'm stingy with the water in this recipe because I don't like waterlogging the squash.)

gingery steamed kabocha squash

1 cup water

2 pounds kabocha or delicata squash, peeled if
    not organic, seeded, and cut into 1½-inch chunks

2 tablespoons minced fresh ginger

prep: about 10 minutes
cooking: 10 to 15 minutes

In a large heavy saucepan, begin bringing the water to a boil. As the water heats, layer the squash (skin side down if unpeeled) in the pan, sprinkling with the ginger as you go. Once the water has come to a boil, cover and cook over medium-high heat until the squash can easily be pierced with a fork, 10 to 15 minutes.

makes 4 servings

a breakfast mix

What ever happened to breakfast? Sometimes the taste of waffles, French toast, and porridge seems to exist only in memory.

In an effort to bring some variety and carefree good cheer to the first meal of the day, I've included a handful of quick vegan versions of some old favorites—plus a few tasty toppings for special occasions. To speed up preparation, I've created quick mixes for waffles and scones.

No need to wait for Sunday morning or a company brunch to have a breakfast that's short on prep and long on pleasure.

unlimited waffle mix

I hadn't had waffles since I was a kid, when most suburban moms (including mine) had newfangled—but certainly not nonstick—electric waffle irons. Now that nonstick surfaces offer fuss-free waffle making, I can enjoy this elegant and easy treat on weekday mornings—especially having made the discovery that an egg-free, whole-grain batter could produce such good taste and crispy texture. (Pancakes made without eggs are another story entirely.)

Preparing several batches of a homemade mix for waffles is not only a healthful alternative to most store-bought mixes, but also a great economy of time and money. I've designed this recipe so that you can measure as many individual batches as you like into small Ziploc freezer bags. Label the bags and keep them in the freezer for up to four months.

basic waffle mix

1 cup whole wheat pastry flour

⅓ cup oat bran

2 teaspoons baking powder

1 teaspoon ground cinnamon

½ teaspoon salt

prep: under 10 minutes (mix)
under 5 minutes (waffles)
cooking: 2 to 3 minutes per waffle

For each batch, measure the ingredients into a small Ziploc freezer bag. Make as many batches as you like. Seal tightly, label, and store the bags in the freezer until needed, up to 4 months.

fruity waffles: Add 3 tablespoons dried currants or minced dried apples, apricots, or pears to the basic mix.

sunflower seed waffles: Add 3 tablespoons raw or toasted sunflower seeds to the basic mix.

to prepare each batch of waffles

Vegetable oil cooking spray

1 to 1¼ cups soy milk

1 tablespoon canola oil

1 tablespoon pure maple syrup

1 batch Basic Waffle Mix

Lightly mist an unheated nonstick waffle iron with vegetable cooking spray. Plug in and heat.

In a 4-cup glass measuring cup, combine 1 cup soy milk with the oil and syrup. Sprinkle in the waffle mix while stirring with a fork. Stir just until blended into a thick batter. If the mixture is too thick to stir or if it thickens on standing, stir in extra soy milk by the tablespoon.

When the waffle iron is hot, spoon in enough batter to cover about three quarters of the surface, leaving the edges of the waffle iron exposed. Close and bake until steam is no longer coming out of the iron and the waffle is crispy, 2 to 3 minutes. Remove and serve immediately, or reserve in a warm place, such as a toaster oven set to 200 degrees, while you cook the remaining waffles.

makes five to six 4-inch Belgian waffles or three 7-inch round waffles

repeat performances You can refrigerate any extra batter overnight. It will thicken considerably; thin to the proper pouring consistency with soy milk. Waffles freeze and reheat beautifully. Wrap them well, label, and freeze for up to 2 months. Reheat the frozen waffles in a toaster oven or a regular toaster.

Serve the waffles for breakfast, piping hot, with your favorite topping: maple syrup, Pear, Currant, and Almond Conserve (page 137), Mango Sauce (page 135), or chopped fresh fruit—or even Cashew Cream (page 132).

For dessert, make waffle sandwiches, filled with your favorite frozen sorbet.

These delightful whole-grain versions of a classic teatime favorite were developed by my able assistant, Rosemary Serviss. With bags of mix ready and waiting in the freezer, it's a snap to prepare freshly baked scones on impulse. The three versions that Rosemary created—walnut, apricot-lemon, and apple-spice—are ideal to serve for breakfast or brunch.

Scones are best when just baked and still warm, but they also freeze beautifully. To defrost and reheat, pop them, still frozen and uncovered, into a preheated 350-degree oven (the toaster oven is convenient) until they are warmed through and crispy on the outside.

For a light texture, be sure to use whole wheat pastry flour, not the kind used for baking bread. Try King Arthur's Round Table flour (a type of whole wheat

super scones

super scone mix

1 cup unbleached all-purpose flour

1 cup whole wheat pastry flour

¼ cup maple sprinkles, Sucanat™, or sugar

2 teaspoons baking powder

½ teaspoon baking soda

½ teaspoon salt

prep: under 10 minutes (mix)
about 15 minutes (scones)

baking: about 15 minutes

For each batch, measure the ingredients into a small Ziploc freezer bag. Seal tightly, label, and store in the freezer until needed, up to 4 months.

walnut scones

1 tablespoon cider vinegar

Approximately ⅔ cup soy milk

2 teaspoons vanilla extract

1 batch Super Scone Mix

⅓ cup Spectrum Spread (see Note)

½ cup toasted walnuts, coarsely chopped

apricot-lemon scones

1 tablespoon freshly squeezed lemon juice

Approximately ⅔ cup soy milk

1 teaspoon vanilla extract

1 batch Super Scone Mix

⅓ cup Spectrum Spread (see Note)

2 tablespoons finely chopped or grated lemon zest (from 2 large lemons, preferably organic)

½ cup chopped dried apricots

apple-spice scones

- 1 tablespoon cider vinegar
- Approximately ⅔ cup soy milk
- 1 teaspoon vanilla extract
- 1 batch Super Scone mix
- 1 teaspoon ground cinnamon
- 1 teaspoon ground ginger
- 1 teaspoon ground mustard
- ½ teaspoon ground cloves
- ⅓ cup Spectrum Spread (see Note)
- 1 large Granny Smith apple, peeled, cored, and finely chopped (about 1 cup)
- ¼ cup dried currants

making the scones

Set the rack in the middle of the oven. Preheat the oven to 425 degrees. Line a cookie sheet with parchment paper (or lightly mist a nonstick cookie sheet with vegetable oil cooking spray).

To make any one of the three recipes, place the cider vinegar or lemon juice in a 1-cup glass measuring cup and add enough soy milk to equal ⅔ cup. Stir in the vanilla extract and set aside. (Don't be alarmed when the mixture curdles; that's what is intended.)

Place the scone mix in a large bowl. If making the apple-spice variation, add the spices. Stir well with a whisk or fork.

Using a table knife, slice off tiny bits of the Spectrum Spread, distributing evenly over the flour mixture. With a pastry blender, cut in the spread until the mixture resembles coarse crumbs. Stir in the remaining ingredients (except the reserved soy milk mixture).

pastry flour; see Mail-Order Sources, page 157) and you'll be hooked on the exceptionally good taste and light texture it produces.

This recipe calls for Spectrum Spread, a nonhydrogenated vegetable shortening that gives the scones a crumbly texture. It's easiest to cut the Spectrum Spread into the flour with a pastry cutter; if you don't own one, use two knives or your fingers. For optimum taste, use full-fat soy milk (not "lite," which is diluted with water).

To eliminate cleanup, line the cookie sheet with baking parchment rather than greasing it.

continued

Drizzle a generous ½ cup of the soy milk mixture over the dry ingredients. Stir with a fork, drizzling on additional soy milk if needed, just until the mixture forms a soft dough.

Divide the dough in half. Place one half on a lightly floured board and, with lightly floured hands, pat into a ¾-inch-thick round. Cut the dough into 6 wedges. Gently separate the wedges and transfer them to the prepared baking sheet. Repeat with remaining dough.

Bake until the tops have a hint of color and the bottoms are lightly browned, 14 to 15 minutes. Transfer the scones to a wire rack. Cool until just warm and serve.

note: Spectrum Spread is available in the refrigerated section of health food stores.

makes 12 scones

cashew cream

½ cup unsalted raw cashews

¼ cup plus 2 tablespoons unflavored soy milk

prep: about 5 minutes

In a blender, process the cashews and soy milk until very smooth, 2 to 3 minutes, stopping once or twice to scrape down the inside of the blender bowl. Refrigerate until needed, up to 3 days.

makes about ½ cup

This luscious spread is a delightful cholesterol-free alternative to clotted cream, the traditional British accompaniment to scones.

Once refrigerated, the mixture will thicken slightly but will remain spreadable. If you wish, thin it slightly by stirring in a few additional teaspoons of soy milk. (Don't be tempted to use reduced-fat soy milk in this recipe; the consistency will be watery.)

smoky tempeh patties

8 ounces tempeh (soy or three-grain),
    cut into 4 to 5 pieces

2 tablespoons water

1 tablespoon canola oil

2 teaspoons dried sage

1 teaspoon Italian Herb Blend (page 16 or store-bought)

¾ teaspoon salt

¼ teaspoon Liquid Smoke

1 large clove garlic

¼ teaspoon crushed red pepper flakes

⅛ teaspoon freshly ground black pepper

Vegetable oil cooking spray

prep: 10 minutes
cooking: 15 minutes steaming,
plus 8 to 10 minutes frying

Pour 2 cups of water into a large saucepan fitted with a steaming basket. Add the tempeh, cover tightly, and steam over medium-high heat for 15 minutes. Transfer the tempeh to the bowl of a food processor and add all the remaining ingredients. Process until the ingredients are well blended and the mixture begins to hold together, about 1 minute, scraping down the bowl once or twice.

For each sausage, shape 2 tablespoons of the mixture into a patty about 2 inches in diameter and ½ inch thick. Set aside on a plate.

Lightly mist a large nonstick skillet or griddle with oil and heat until hot. Place as many patties as will fit in one layer in the skillet, and immediately flip them over (this is done to lightly coat the surface with oil). Cook over medium heat, covered, until light brown on the underside, 3 to 5 minutes. Flip over, cover, and brown on the second side, 2 to 3 minutes. Drain on paper towels and repeat with any remaining patties. Serve hot.

makes eight 2-inch patties

These breakfast patties are made with tempeh, a dense fermented soybean cake available in the refrigerated section of health food stores. Adding herbs—and the smoke flavor associated with traditional sausage—gives them a homey, familiar taste. I much prefer these to the purchased soy-based sausages I've tried. Don't be tempted to eliminate the tablespoon of oil in the recipe; it's needed for texture and to bind the mixture. The finished patties can be kept warm in a 200-degree oven until ready to serve, up to fifteen minutes. Cooked patties may be frozen for up to one month.

banana french toast

This is a very simple, tasty, dairy-free French toast, in which bananas make a surprising appearance as a substitute for the traditional eggs. Serve for brunch with a variety of homemade toppings and Smoky Tempeh Patties (page 133).

For best results, use a nonstick griddle or skillet. (The sugars in the bananas have a tendency to burn; for this reason, cast-iron griddles don't work with this recipe!) Get the griddle good and hot before adding the dipped bread, and allow any excess batter to drip off the bread before cooking. Alternatively, bake the French toast on a nonstick cookie sheet at 400 degrees until browned on the bottom, fifteen to twenty minutes. Serve with the browned sides up.

2 cups sliced bananas (2 medium bananas)

¾ cup vanilla soy milk

1 teaspoon ground cinnamon

8 slices day-old whole wheat or sourdough bread

Vegetable oil cooking spray

Mango Sauce (page 135), Pear, Currant, and Almond Conserve (page 137), maple syrup, or fruit-sweetened jam

prep: 10 minutes
cooking: 5 minutes per batch

Place the bananas, soy milk, and cinnamon in a blender or food processor and blend until smooth. Pour the mixture into a pie plate. Dip a slice of bread into the mixture. Prick a few times with a fork to encourage absorption. Turn to coat the second side. Let excess batter drip off, and set aside on a large plate. Repeat with the remaining slices.

Mist a large nonstick griddle or skillet with the cooking spray and heat until very hot. With a spatula, lift the dipped bread and transfer it to the griddle. Cook (in batches if necessary) over medium-high heat until browned on the bottom, 2 to 3 minutes. Flip over and brown the second side. Transfer to warm plates and serve immediately, accompanied with your favorite topping.

makes 8 slices

mango sauce

1 ripe mango

prep: 5 minutes

Peel the mango (an ordinary peeler does the job nicely) and slice the flesh away from the large pit. Discard the pit and cut the flesh into large chunks. Puree the flesh in a blender or food processor. Transfer to a bowl and serve immediately.

makes about 1 cup

When mangoes are in season, serve this puree instead of maple syrup as a topping for waffles or French toast. It tastes best when freshly prepared and made with a room-temperature mango—otherwise, you'll be putting an ice-cold topping on your piping-hot breakfast.

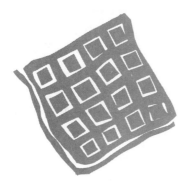

Here's a nice way to fill up on the wholesome goodness of rolled oats without turning on the stove. The oats "cook" overnight in the refrigerator as they soak in unsweetened pineapple juice and rice milk.

I like to prepare this breakfast during the summer, when I want to keep both the kitchen and myself cool. If you wish, top the chilled oatmeal with more fresh fruit in season, such as strawberries, blueberries, or sliced peaches.

overnight pineapple oats

2 cups old-fashioned rolled oats

1 (8-ounce) can unsweetened crushed pineapple

1½ cups rice or soy milk

¼ to ½ teaspoon ground cardamom

⅛ teaspoon salt

1 to 2 ripe bananas, sliced

¼ cup chopped toasted nuts, sunflower seeds, or untoasted ground flax seeds

prep: 5 minutes
standing: overnight refrigeration

In a medium glass bowl or nonreactive storage container, combine the oats, pineapple, rice milk, cardamom, and salt. Stir well, cover, and refrigerate overnight.

In the morning, stir in the sliced bananas. Divide evenly among four bowls and top each serving with 1 tablespoon toasted nuts.

makes 4 servings

whole grains for breakfast

Wake up to a freshly cooked batch of whole grains for breakfast. The night before, cook kamut, wheat berries, brown rice, or spelt (or a combination) with a dash of cinnamon in a slow cooker (set on Low, if you have a choice); use 2 cups of water for each cup of dry grain. In the morning, stir in raisins or sliced fresh fruit and add maple syrup to taste.

pear, currant, and almond conserve

2 cups peeled, cored, and finely diced Bosc or
    Anjou pears (3 medium pears)

¼ cup dried currants, cherries, or blueberries

3 tablespoons Amaretto, Grand Marnier, or Cointreau liqueur

½ teaspoon ground cinnamon

⅛ teaspoon ground cardamom or freshly grated nutmeg (optional)

2 tablespoons slivered almonds

prep: 10 minutes

cooking: about 10 minutes

In a heavy saucepan, combine the pears, currants, Amaretto, cinnamon, and cardamom (if using). Bring to a boil over high heat. Reduce the heat to low and simmer, uncovered, stirring occasionally, until the pears are tender, about 10 minutes. Stir in the almonds. Cool to room temperature.

Transfer the conserve to a jar and refrigerate until needed.

makes about 1 cup

This is an unusually delicious, chunky topping for your breakfast toast, waffles, or French toast. The only constants are the pears, almonds, and cinnamon. Otherwise, have fun varying the dried fruit, spices, and liqueur. The conserve may be refrigerated in a tightly sealed jar for up to one month.

For optimum flavor, use ripe pears.

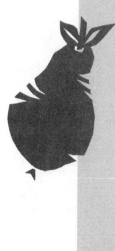

fuss-free desserts

Like many people, I'm often in the mood for a little something sweet at the end of the meal. But I rarely get around to preparing anything unless company is coming. This is a shame, because dessert is surely one of life's simple pleasures—cool ices, warm crisps, crunchy cookies, chewy apricot confections—and those pleasures can be a treat every day with very little extra effort.

For those of you who join me in wanting to enjoy dessert a bit more often, I've designed some fuss-free recipes to satisfy that desire. There's a mix to please the cookie monster and other recipes that can be made ahead and refrigerated or frozen—ready and waiting for that moment when your sweet tooth prevails.

crispy cookie mix

½ cup old-fashioned rolled oats

½ cup unblanched whole almonds

½ cup whole wheat pastry flour

¼ teaspoon salt

prep: 10 minutes (mix)
15 minutes (cookies)

baking: about 15 minutes

In a food processor fitted with the metal blade, combine all ingredients and pulse until the oats and almonds are coarsely ground. Transfer to a Ziploc freezer bag. Label, seal tightly, and store in the freezer until needed, up to 4 months.

almond cookies

¼ cup canola oil

¼ cup pure maple syrup

1½ teaspoons vanilla extract

¼ teaspoon almond extract

1 batch Crispy Cookie Mix

oatmeal chip cookies

¼ cup canola oil

¼ cup pure maple syrup

1 teaspoon vanilla extract

1 batch Crispy Cookie Mix

½ cup chocolate chips (malt-sweetened are nice)

oatmeal raisin spice cookies

¼ cup canola oil

¼ cup pure maple syrup

1 teaspoon vanilla extract

1 batch Crispy Cookie Mix

There's nothing quite like the sweet smell of cookies baking in the oven, or the pleasure of eating them while they're still warm. I am really sold on the idea of homemade baking mixes, because they make it so easy to whip up a batch of cookies spontaneously. I offer three variations on the basic mix, and I'd be hard put to tell you which one I like best.

If you want to make several batches of mix at a time, prepare each separately to insure accurate measures of the ingredients.

⅓ cup raisins

½ teaspoon ground cinnamon

¼ teaspoon freshly grated nutmeg

making the cookies

Position the oven rack in the middle of the oven and preheat the oven to 375 degrees. For easy cleanup, line a cookie sheet with baking parchment. Otherwise, use a nonstick cookie sheet or lightly grease a standard cookie sheet.

To make any one of the three recipes, in a glass measuring cup, whisk together the liquid ingredients until thoroughly blended. Pour the cookie mix into a medium bowl and stir in any remaining dry ingredients. Make a well in the center of the dry ingredients, add the liquid, and stir with a fork to combine. Do not overmix.

Drop level tablespoonfuls of the dough onto the prepared cookie sheet. With your fingers, flatten each mound of dough into a disc about ⅓ inch thick.

Bake the cookies until golden on the bottom, 13 to 15 minutes. With a spatula, remove from the cookie sheet and cool on a wire rack. Refrigerate in an airtight container for up to 1 week, or freeze for up to 2 months.

makes about 20 cookies

apricot-walnut balls

¾ cup loosely packed apricots, preferably
   unsulphured

⅓ cup walnuts

1 teaspoon anise seeds

¼ cup unsweetened dried grated coconut

prep: about 15 minutes

In a food processor, combine the apricots, walnuts, and anise seeds. Process until the apricots and nuts are finely chopped and begin to clump together.

Spread the coconut out on a plate. Shape rounded teaspoonfuls of the apricot mixture into small balls, rolling them between your palms. Roll the balls in the coconut and place in an airtight container. Refrigerate until needed, up to 1 month.

makes 17 to 18 balls

tropical fruit crisp

1 (20-ounce) can unsweetened pineapple
    chunks, drained (juice reserved)

2 large ripe bananas, halved lengthwise and
    cut into 1/2-inch chunks

2 tablespoons unsweetened, dried, grated coconut

1/2 teaspoon ground cinnamon

Large pinch of freshly grated nutmeg

1/4 cup reserved pineapple juice or 2 tablespoons pineapple juice and
    2 tablespoons light rum

1 1/2 cups of your favorite granola

prep: under 10 minutes
baking: 25 minutes

Position the rack in the center of the oven and preheat the oven to 350 degrees.

In an 8-inch square glass baking dish, combine the pineapple and bananas. Sprinkle with the coconut, cinnamon, and nutmeg and toss to blend. Pour the pineapple juice (and the rum, if using) over the fruit. Sprinkle the granola over the top.

Bake, uncovered, for 25 minutes. Serve warm.

note: Leftovers can be refrigerated for up to 3 days. The bananas will turn brown, but the crisp will still taste good.

makes 4 to 6 servings

This homey crisp is full of intriguing flavors and textures. Thanks to the use of store-bought granola for the topping, it can be thrown together in no time. I prefer granola that has walnuts and raisins tossed in, but you can use the "no-fat-added" variety if you prefer.

I think you will be delighted—as I was—to discover the rich taste and creamy texture of baked bananas. Serve them crisp warm from the oven, topped perhaps with a scoop of mango or coconut sorbet.

pineapple-ginger ice

I large ripe pineapple

I to I ½ tablespoons finely minced or grated fresh ginger (depending upon your love of the flavor)

Pure maple syrup to taste (optional)

Fresh mint leaves for garnish (optional)

prep: 10 minutes

freezing: at least 2 to 3 hours

Cut off the top and slice the pineapple lengthwise into quarters. Slice off the sliver of hard core from each quarter. With a serrated knife, using a sawing motion, slice the skin from the flesh. Cut each pineapple quarter into thin slices. Place the slices in a tightly sealed container or Ziploc bag and freeze for 2 to 3 hours (or longer, if convenient).

About 15 minutes before serving, remove the pineapple from the freezer. Just before serving, break up the frozen pineapple slices and pulse them with the ginger in a food processor until the fruit is finely chopped. If you wish, add enough maple syrup to sweeten and heighten the flavors and pulse once or twice more. Serve immediately in chilled small bowls or parfait glasses, garnished with mint leaves, if you wish.

note: Ripe pineapples are a rich golden brown, yield slightly when squeezed, and have a sweet aroma most detectable at the base. If you pull a leaf from the crown, it should come out easily.

makes 4 to 6 servings

carefree any-fruit granita

2 cups bottled fruit juice (one fruit or a blend)

prep: 1 minute
freezing: 2 to 3 hours

Pour the juice into a standard ice cube tray. Freeze until firm, 2 to 3 hours.

Transfer the frozen cubes to the bowl of a food processor fitted with the metal blade, and pulse until slushy. Serve immediately in chilled small bowls or parfait glasses.

makes 4 servings

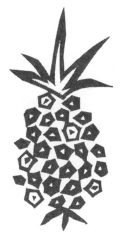

Fruit juices freeze beautifully and make very refreshing and healthful ices. Making this granita is almost as easy as making ice cubes!

There is such a vast array of berry and exotic fruit juice blends available nowadays that you can enjoy a different type of frozen fruit just about every week. Pomegranate and mango are two of my favorites.

For a richer, more sherbetlike consistency, substitute coconut milk for half a cup of your chosen tropical fruit juice and blend thoroughly before freezing.

Frozen ripe bananas and strawberries pureed together become a remarkably creamy dessert, with a richness reminiscent of old-fashioned sherbet. Layering the mélange with fresh berries makes a very attractive parfait and a refreshing finale to a spicy meal.

You can buy the strawberries already frozen, either whole or sliced. (Some cooks consider frozen fruits inferior. However, organic frozen fruits, having been picked and frozen at the height of their flavor, are usually excellent.) Or, trim and halve some fresh strawberries and freeze them yourself. Consider the amount of fruit as a rule of thumb; a little more or less doesn't matter.

Timing counts: Barely defrost the fruits, for about five minutes only, before pureeing, then serve the parfait immediately after you've assembled it.

frozen berry parfaits

I large ripe banana, peeled, sliced, and frozen

I cup frozen whole or sliced strawberries

½ cup soy or rice milk

¼ teaspoon ground cardamom

Pure maple syrup to taste

¾ cup fresh blueberries, raspberries, or blackberries

prep: 5 minutes
(assuming already-frozen fruit)

About 10 minutes before you plan to serve the dessert, remove the fruit from the freezer and allow it to stand at room temperature for about 5 minutes. Place the banana slices, strawberries, soy milk, and cardamom in the bowl of a food processor or blender and process until smooth. Taste and add maple syrup as needed, then pulse once or twice to blend.

Place a dollop of the frozen puree in the bottom of three chilled parfait glasses or small bowls. Spoon some berries on top, and continue alternating frozen puree and berries. Serve immediately.

makes 3 servings

peaches with fresh blueberry sauce

1 pint fresh blueberries

prep: 10 minutes

1 to 2 teaspoons finely minced or grated lemon
   zest, preferably from an organic lemon

Pure maple syrup to taste

4 large ripe peaches, peeled (if desired) and sliced

Fresh mint leaves for garnish

Puree the blueberries in a blender or food processor. Blend in the lemon zest and maple syrup to taste. Make a puddle of the sauce on each dessert plate, and fan out the peach slices, overlapping them slightly, on top. Garnish with fresh mint leaves.

makes 4 servings

Most of the work involved in this memorable but minimalist dessert is in finding the best peaches and blueberries available.

ingredients at a glance

Here's a handy reference list describing many of the ingredients in this book, with an emphasis on the nonperishable items. (For guidance on fresh vegetable preparation, see pages 8–10.)

In many cases, I've recommended specific brands when I've used them particularly successfully in recipe testing or found them to be superior. "Other Good Choices" offer you alternatives, and of course you may already have some favorite brands of your own. When there are no specific recommendations, I haven't found dramatic variations among brands I've tried. In a few instances, when I felt it would be useful, I've offered storage advice too.

Anything in this list that is not sold in your local supermarket or gourmet shop should be available in any well-stocked natural food store. If you are fortunate enough to live near a large natural food supermarket like Wild Oats or Whole Foods, you'll have the convenience of one-stop shopping. If you're eager to try recommended brands but can't find them, ask the store manager to place a special order with his distributor.

All items of Asian origin—such as pickled ginger and toasted sesame oil—are also sold in Asian markets. I've recommended Mail-Order Sources (see page 156) for less common ingredients and for specialty items of superior quality.

arame: A mild-flavored slightly briny sea vegetable whose wide leaves are finely shredded, precooked, and sun-dried. It's ready to eat after a brief soak in ample water to cover.

balsamic vinegar: Wine vinegar from Modena, Italy, which, at its best, has a syrupy texture and mild sweetness. Recommended Brand: Cavalli. Mail-Order Source: Dean & DeLuca. If using supermarket brands, which are more acidic, add with caution, beginning with the minimum amount called for in the recipe.

barley: See quick-cooking barley.

basil olive oil: Olive oil infused with the flavor of fresh basil. To make your own, see page 18. Recommended Brand: Consorzio. Mail-Order Source: Dean & DeLuca. Other Good Choices: Boyajian and Loriva. Storage: Refrigerator.

black (brown) mustard seeds: A spice commonly used in Indian cooking; develops a nutty flavor when sizzled and popped in oil. Available in Indian markets. Mail-Order Source: Adriana's Caravan.

black soybeans: A dark-skinned variety of soybean, these are renowned for their creamy texture and delicate "chestnutty" taste. Mail-Order Source (dried): Goldmine. Recommended Brand (canned): Eden.

brown rice, quick™: A precooked brown rice that is ready to eat in about twelve minutes. Recommended Brand: Arrowhead Mills.

brown-rice udon: A whole-grain noodle made from a combination of brown rice and whole wheat flours; cooks in only five to seven minutes. Recommended Brand: Eden Foods. Storage: Refrigerator.

brown rice vinegar: Mild, full-bodied, slightly sweet fermented vinegar made from cooked brown rice.

chili powder: A blend of chili peppers, cumin, oregano, and other flavorings; try a few brands until you find a blend and "heat" you like. Recommended Brand: Spice Garden (Spike brand). Mail-Order Source: Adriana's Caravan (offers a large variety).

chipotle chili powder: Finely ground dried stemmed and seeded chipotle chilies; lends a smoky flavor to any dish. It's easy to make your own in a spice grinder. (Remove stems and discard seeds.) Can be very hot, so use with discretion. Mail-Order Sources: Los Chileros de New Mexico and King Arthur.

coconut (unsweetened, dried, grated): Readily available in health food stores and Indian groceries; it is often called "desiccated." (Just make sure no sugar has been added.) If only flaked coconut is available, finely chop it in a food processor fitted with the metal blade. Storage: Freezer.

corn (frozen): Doesn't require cooking; just defrost (rinse under hot water if it's covered with ice crystals). Toss into salads or add at the last minute to cooked dishes. Recommended Brand: Cascadian Farms Organic.

curry blend: A highly variable blend of spices, from hot to mild. Try making your own (page 17). Recommended Brand: Adriana's Caravan Jamaican Curry. Other Good Choices: Frontier Curry Powder and Madras Curry Powder (Merwanjee Poonjiajee & Sons; sold in a tin in many gourmet shops). Mail-Order Source: Adriana's Caravan. Storage: Refrigerator.

diced tomatoes with green chilies: An outstanding organic canned product with vibrant taste; Eden brand is made with Roma tomatoes (skins intact) and jalapeño chilies. Recommended Brand: Eden Foods. Other Good Choices: Del Monte Salsa-Style Tomatoes and Muir Glen Mexican-Style Tomatoes with Chipotles.

dijon mustard: A traditional French mustard made of mustard seeds, vinegar, and white wine. Recommended Brand: Maille.

frozen vegetables: Recommended Brand: Cascadian Farms Organic. Other good choice: Tree of Life.

harissa: A North African hot pepper paste sold in a can or tube in many international groceries. Mail-Order Source: Adriana's Caravan.

herbamare: An imported Swiss seasoning blend of sea salt and organically grown vegetables and herbs; usually available in natural food stores.

herbes de provence: A blend usually containing basil, tarragon, summer savory, rosemary, and marjoram. Make your own (page 17) or purchase. Recommended Brand and Mail-Order Source: Adriana's Caravan.

hot pepper sesame oil: A type of chili oil, this is thick toasted sesame oil flavored with red chili peppers. The "heat" of different brands varies; the recipes in this book have been tested with Eden brand, which is relatively mild. If using another Asian chili oil, add according to taste.

instant beans: Dehydrated and ground cooked, beans that are ready to eat after steeping in boiling water for about five minutes; sometimes seasoned. Recommended Brand: Fantastic Foods Instant Black Beans and Refried Beans.

instant polenta: A precooked cornmeal that takes five minutes or less to cook (adjust timing of recipes for brands that take longer). Recommended Brands: Valsugana and Tipiak.

instant potato flakes: Flaked dried potatoes that reconstitute instantly upon contact with hot water. Recommended Brand: Barbara's.

instant vegetable stock powder: A powdered blend of dehydrated vegetables, herbs, and spices that can be used as a seasoning or reconstituted with water into a stock. Recommended Brand: Vogue Vege Base. Other Good Choices: Morga and Frontier (bulk). Storage: Refrigerator.

instant wakame sea vegetable: Dehydrated mineral-rich flakes that need only brief soaking in liquid; adds a briny flavor to soups and stews. Recommended Brand: Eden Foods.

italian herb blend: An herb mixture usually containing oregano, basil, thyme, rosemary, and (sometimes) fennel seed and crushed red pepper flakes. Make your own (page 16) or purchase. Mail-Order Source: Adriana's Caravan.

japanese-style pickled ginger: See pickled ginger.

kamut: An ancient grain about three times the size of wheat berries, with a buttery taste, chewy texture, and impressive nutritional profile. Available in most health food stores. Mail-Order Source: Goldmine. Storage: Freezer.

lentils (canned): Use either plain or seasoned in these recipes. Recommended Brand: Eden Foods (seasoned).

liquid smoke: A liquid blend of water and mesquite or hickory flavor; very little is needed to impart a strong smoky taste. Available in supermarkets.

maple sprinkles: Dehydrated maple syrup that can be used in baking; also known as maple sugar. Mail-Order Source: Vermont Country Maple.

mesclun: A mix of various baby lettuces and bitter greens, often organic; increasingly available in supermarkets. Storage: Unwashed in a perforated bag in the vegetable bin—use as soon as possible.

mexican-style tomatoes with chipotles: Canned stewed tomatoes flavored with chipotle chilies. Substitute for Eden Food's Diced Tomatoes with Green Chilies if necessary. Recommended Brand: Muir Glen. Other Good Choice: Del Monte Salsa-Style Tomatoes.

miso: A fermented soybean paste with a complex, winy flavor, traditionally used in Japanese cooking. Light misos are generally sweeter and less salty than dark ones; you can enhance flavor by combining two or more types. Look for unpasteurized (refrigerated) varieties in natural food stores. Mail-Order Source: Goldmine.

parmesan cheese: Opt for best-quality Italian Parmigiano-Reggiano. Storage: Refrigerate whole chunk and grate as needed. Or, grate a batch and freeze in a tightly sealed container (this is convenient and little flavor is lost).

pasta sauce: See spaghetti sauce.

pickled ginger: A traditional Japanese product (also known as sushi ginger) prepared by pickling fresh ginger sliced paper-thin in vinegar, salt, and a sweetener. It is available in health food stores, Asian groceries, and many salad bars that have sushi. Recipes in this book have been tested with Japanese pickled ginger, *not* Chinese, which is prepared differently. Recommended Brand: Eden Foods. Storage: Refrigerate in a jar in its own pickling juice.

pickled ginger juice: The intensely ginger-flavored brine in which Japanese pickled ginger is stored.

quick brown rice: See brown rice, quick™.

quick-cooking barley: A precooked barley that is ready to eat in about twelve minutes. Recommended Brand: Mother's (best flavor and texture). Other Good Choice: Quaker.

quinoa: A small, quick-cooking grain native to the Andes; high in protein and easy to digest. Best to buy in sealed bags or boxes. (Avoid buying in bulk unless it is kept refrigerated or your health food store has rapid turnover.) Rinse well (see page 44) to remove the bitter coating. Mail-Order Source: Goldmine. Storage: Freezer.

rice noodles: Also known as *bifun*, *mifun* (rice sticks), and rice vermicelli. A quick-cooking, tasty alternative to wheat pasta.

roasted garlic olive oil: Olive oil infused with the mild flavor of roasted garlic. Recommended Brand: Consorzio. Mail-Order Source: Dean & DeLuca. Some brands of garlic oil use raw garlic and have a much stronger flavor. These are convenient if you plan to cook with them, but for other uses they can be too assertive, and you'll probably want to use a combination of minced fresh garlic and plain olive oil.

roasted red peppers: If you don't feel like making your own (page 9), roasted peppers in a jar are a reasonable substitute. Unless you use them frequently, buy small jars; once opened, they'll last only about two weeks. Storage: Refrigerator.

rosemary olive oil: Olive oil infused with the flavor of fresh rosemary. To make your own, see page 18. Recommended Brand: Consorzio. Mail-Order Source: Dean & DeLuca. Storage: Refrigerator.

salsa: A condiment/dip that usually features tomatoes, chilies, and cilantro. The taste and heat of different brands vary widely. Recommended Brands: Timpone's Salsa Muy Rica and El Paso Chili Company's Chipotle Cha Cha Cha. Other Good Choices: Enrico's and Newman's Own.

sesame tahini: Also called sesame butter; a paste made of ground sesame seeds. Recommended Brand: Joyva (sold in Middle Eastern groceries).

shiitake mushrooms (dried): Also called Chinese black mushrooms. Intensely flavorful Asian mushrooms traditionally grown on oak logs, then dried in the sun. After steeping them in hot water to soften them, trim off the inedible stems (which may be used in making stock). Storage: Cool, dry place.

shoyu: Traditional Japanese soy sauce made of soybeans, wheat, and an enzyme that causes fermentation. Look for brands that don't contain caramel coloring or other additives. Do not substitute Chinese soy sauce, which is considerably saltier. Recommended Brands: Eden Organic Shoyu and Ohsawa Nama Shoyu.

soy milk: A nutrient-rich liquid made by pressing ground, simmered soy beans. It is sold in one-liter shelf-stable aseptic "bricks" and labeled either soy beverage or drink. Recommended Brand: Edensoy Extra Original (fortified).

spaghetti sauce: With so many brands to choose from, it can get confusing. Recommended Brands: Classico and Newman's Own are old reliables.

spectrum spread: A nonhydrogenated, dairy-free solid vegetable shortening made from canola oil and soy protein isolate. Available in the refrigerated section of most natural food stores. Storage: Refrigerator.

sucanat™: Granulated cane juice that retains minerals and trace elements of sugarcane. Sold in health food stores.

tamari: A wheat-free fermented soy sauce made from soybeans, salt, water, and a soy-derived starter called *koji*. Look for brands that don't contain caramel coloring or other additives. Do not substitute Chinese soy sauce, which is much saltier.

tempeh: Fermented soybean cake. Those made with grains rather than all soy have a milder flavor. Storage: Freezer (for longer storage) or refrigerator.

thai red curry paste: A thick curry blend containing red chilies, onions, garlic, spices, and salt (some brands contain dried shrimp); available in cans or jars. Recommended Brand: Thai Kitchen (vegetarian). Storage: Keeps indefinitely in a jar in the refrigerator.

toasted sesame oil: An intensely flavored thick oil extracted from pressed roasted sesame seeds. Recommended Brand: Eden. Storage: Refrigerator. See also hot pepper sesame oil.

tofu: Also known as bean curd. Choose one-pound sealed tubs of organic fresh (refrigerated) firm or extra-firm tofu when making stir-fries. Silken tofu (refrigerated fresh or shelf-stable aseptic-packed) is a convenient choice to keep on hand for dressings. Storage: Refrigerate or freeze fresh tofu (see page 10).

tortillas: Whole wheat tortillas are sold in the refrigerator or freezer section of most supermarkets. Recommended Brand: Garden of Eatin'. Or substitute a similar product called Mountain Bread.

whole wheat couscous: For best value, buy in bulk. Storage: Refrigerator.

whole wheat pastry flour: Ground from a variety of wheat that is low in gluten. Mail-Order Source: For a whole wheat pastry flour that produces lighter, sweeter baked goods than most brands, order Round Table flour from King Arthur.

mail-order sources

Most of the sources listed below offer catalogues free or for a nominal charge.

Adriana's Caravan
800-316-0820
One-stop shopping for the best in ethnic condiments and seasonings, including high-quality dried herbs and spices and top-notch infused oils from a variety of makers.

Dean & DeLuca
800-221–7714
A wide range of gourmet food items, including Consorzio infused oils.

El Paso Chile Company
800-27-IS-HOT
A delightful selection of the company's own salsas, bean dips, and hot sauces.

Goldmine Natural Food Company

800-475-3663

A highly recommended source for top-quality organic ingredients, including superior whole grains and superb unpasteurized misos.

Indian Harvest

800-294-2433

A fine selection of exotic grain blends and heirloom dried beans.

King Arthur Flour Baker's Catalogue

800-827-6836

An extensive selection of baking equipment, specialty flours (including Round Table whole wheat pastry flour), and extracts (many organic). Also sells ground chipotles.

Loriva

800-94-LORIVA

A wide range of infused oils. Try especially the intense peanut oil and delicious roasted nut oils.

Los Chileros de Nuevo Mexico

505-471-6967

Excellent source of dried chili peppers, including chipotles and chipotle powder.

Timpone's Fresh Food Corporation

800-883-3238

Great-tasting Salsa Muy Rica and Classic Spaghetti Sauce.

Vermont Country Maple

802-864-7519 or 800-528-7021

A good source of maple sprinkles (maple sugar) at a reasonable price.

Zabar's

212-787-2000 or 800-697-6301

Cookware (including pressure cookers) at discount prices.

index